TRANSLATIONAL MEDICINE

From Discovery to Patient Care

Dr Essam abdelhakim

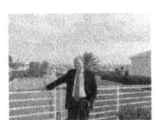

Copyright © 2024 Dr Essam Abdelhakim

All rights reserved

The characters and events portrayed in this book are fictitious. Any similarity to real persons, living or dead, is coincidental and not intended by the author.

No part of this book may be reproduced, or stored in a retrieval system, or transmitted in any form or by any means, electronic, mechanical, photocopying, recording, or otherwise, without express written permission of the publisher.

Cover design by: Art Painter
Library of Congress Control Number: 2018675309
Printed in the United States of America

CONTENTS

Title Page
Copyright
Introduction — 1
Part I: Foundations of Translational Medicine — 5
Chapter 1: Understanding Translational Research — 6
Chapter 2: The Research-to-Patient Pipeline — 12
Chapter 3: Ethical Considerations — 19
Part II: Key Components and Stakeholders — 24
Chapter 4: Collaborations in Translational Medicine — 25
Chapter 5: Role of Technology and Innovation — 29
Chapter 6: Regulatory Pathways — 34
Chapter 7: Bridging the Research Funding Gap — 42
Chapter 8: Overcoming Barriers in Implementation — 50
Chapter 9: Data Management and Sharing — 59
Chapter 10: Translational Medicine in Oncology — 66
Chapter 11: Translational Medicine in Rare Diseases — 73
Chapter 12: Translational Medicine in Infectious Diseases — 79
Chapter 13: Emerging Trends in Translational Medicine — 86
Chapter 14: Building a Sustainable Future — 93
Chapter 15: Conclusion and Call to Action — 100
Appendix — 106

About The Author

INTRODUCTION

Definition and Importance of Translational Medicine

Translational medicine, often referred to as "bench-to-bedside" research, is the process of applying findings from basic scientific research to clinical and community settings to improve health outcomes.

It is a multidisciplinary field that bridges the gap between laboratory discoveries and real-world patient care. This integration involves not only scientific rigor but also collaboration across diverse domains, including clinical research, policy-making, industry, and patient advocacy.

The importance of translational medicine lies in its ability to accelerate the development of diagnostic tools, therapies, and preventive strategies.

By focusing on practical applications of research, translational medicine addresses critical gaps, such as the lag between scientific discoveries and their implementation in healthcare.

It enables the seamless transformation of promising concepts into tangible medical interventions that can improve the quality of life, reduce disease burden, and enhance healthcare systems globally.

Key Benefits Of Translational Medicine Include:

1. **Improved Patient Outcomes:** By prioritizing patient-centric approaches, translational medicine ensures that scientific advancements translate into accessible and effective treatments.
2. **Enhanced Collaboration:** It fosters communication

and partnerships between scientists, clinicians, industry leaders, and policymakers, creating a holistic healthcare innovation ecosystem.
3. **Economic Impact:** Translational medicine reduces waste in research by focusing on practical and impactful projects, which can lower healthcare costs and promote efficient resource allocation.

History And Evolution Of Translational Medicine

The concept of translational medicine has deep historical roots, dating back to the early 20th century. However, its formal recognition as a distinct discipline is relatively recent.

1. **Early Beginnings:**
   In the 19th and early 20th centuries, figures such as Louis Pasteur demonstrated the potential of translational research by applying laboratory discoveries to combat diseases like rabies. Similarly, the discovery of antibiotics like penicillin in the 1920s exemplified how basic research could revolutionize medical care.
2. **Mid-20th Century Advances:**
   The mid-1900s saw significant breakthroughs, such as the development of vaccines and chemotherapies. However, there was limited structured collaboration between laboratory researchers and clinicians, leading to delays in implementing these advances in practice.
3. **The Emergence of Translational Medicine:**
   By the late 20th century, the biomedical community recognized the need for systematic frameworks to ensure that research findings directly benefited patients. This led to the emergence of translational research programs, particularly in the United States and Europe, often supported by government funding

and institutional initiatives.

4. **Modern Era:**
   In the 21st century, translational medicine has become a cornerstone of healthcare innovation. Advances in genomics, bioinformatics, and personalized medicine have fueled its growth. High-profile global initiatives like the Human Genome Project and the Cancer Moonshot Program embody the spirit of translational medicine by combining cutting-edge research with actionable healthcare solutions.

Scope And Applications In Modern Healthcare

The scope of translational medicine is vast, encompassing a wide array of scientific disciplines and medical specialties.
It is instrumental in addressing some of the most pressing challenges in healthcare today.

1. **Diagnostics and Biomarkers:**
   Translational research plays a crucial role in developing diagnostic tools and biomarkers that enable early disease detection, prognosis, and treatment monitoring. For instance, the use of liquid biopsies for cancer detection has revolutionized oncology diagnostics.

2. **Therapeutics:**
   Translational medicine accelerates the discovery and application of novel therapeutics. From targeted cancer therapies like CAR-T cells to gene editing technologies like CRISPR, translational approaches have been pivotal in bringing advanced treatments to patients.

3. **Personalized Medicine:**
   By leveraging genetic, proteomic, and metabolomic data, translational medicine enables the development

of personalized treatment plans tailored to individual patients, thereby improving efficacy and reducing side effects.

4. **Public Health Applications:**
   Translational medicine extends beyond individual patient care to influence population health. For example, vaccine development for infectious diseases such as COVID-19 illustrates the rapid application of research findings to global public health challenges.

5. **Addressing Rare Diseases:**
   Many rare diseases lack effective treatments due to limited research funding and resources. Translational medicine provides a framework to prioritize these conditions, resulting in significant advancements in orphan drug development and innovative therapies.

6. **Health Systems and Policy:**
   Translational medicine informs evidence-based policymaking by providing actionable insights from research. This ensures that health systems are designed to incorporate the latest scientific knowledge into routine care.

PART I: FOUNDATIONS OF TRANSLATIONAL MEDICINE

CHAPTER 1: UNDERSTANDING TRANSLATIONAL RESEARCH

Overview Of Translational Research Phases (T0-T4)

Translational research is often conceptualized as a continuum comprising five distinct phases (T0–T4), each representing a crucial step in bridging basic research and real-world patient care. *These phases* guide the systematic progression of knowledge from the laboratory to societal health impact.

T0: Basic Research

- **Focus:** Foundational studies to explore disease mechanisms at molecular, cellular, or genetic levels.
- **Activities:** Discovery of potential drug targets, understanding pathophysiology, and identifying biomarkers.
- **Output:** Hypotheses, proof-of-concept studies, and preclinical data.
- **Example:** Identification of HER2 gene overexpression in breast cancer, laying the groundwork for targeted therapy.

T1: Translation To Humans

- **Focus:** Transitioning from preclinical studies to first-in-human trials.

- **Activities:** Phase I clinical trials to test safety, dosing, and pharmacokinetics of interventions.
- **Output:** Validation of concepts in humans and determination of safety profiles.
- **Example:** Testing the safety of mRNA vaccine technology in early-stage clinical trials.

T2: Translation To Patients

- **Focus:** Determining the efficacy and clinical utility of interventions.
- **Activities:** Phase II and III clinical trials, development of clinical guidelines, and regulatory approval processes.
- **Output:** Evidence-based treatments and approval for routine clinical use.
- **Example:** Clinical trials demonstrating the efficacy of CAR-T cell therapy for leukemia.

T3: Translation To Practice

- **Focus:** Implementing evidence-based interventions in real-world healthcare settings.
- **Activities:** Health services research, quality improvement projects, and integration into clinical workflows.
- **Output:** Improved patient outcomes and healthcare practices.
- **Example:** Introduction of electronic prescribing systems to reduce medication errors.

T4: Translation To Population Health

- **Focus:** Evaluating the broader impact of interventions on public health.
- **Activities:** Epidemiological studies, policy analysis, and health economic evaluations.
- **Output:** Population-level health improvements and policy recommendations.
- **Example:** Widespread adoption of the HPV vaccine to reduce cervical cancer rates globally.

Differences Between Basic, Clinical, And Translational Research

1. Basic Research:
- **Purpose:** To explore fundamental biological processes and uncover new knowledge.
- **Setting:** Laboratory-based, using in vitro (e.g., cell cultures) or in vivo (e.g., animal models) studies.
- **Output:** Theoretical insights and identification of potential therapeutic targets.
- **Example:** Mapping the structure of a viral protein to understand its role in infection.

2. Clinical Research:
- **Purpose:** To study interventions in humans to determine their safety, efficacy, and outcomes.
- **Setting:** Conducted in clinical environments such as hospitals or research centers.
- **Output:** Data supporting clinical decision-making and regulatory approval.
- **Example:** Phase II trial testing a new diabetes medication in patients.

3. Translational Research:
- **Purpose:** To bridge the gap between basic and clinical research by ensuring that discoveries lead to practical applications.
- **Setting:** Involves collaboration across laboratories, clinics, and healthcare systems.
- **Output:** Interventions that are ready for widespread clinical use and public health implementation.
- **Example:** Developing a drug delivery system based on nanotechnology to improve cancer treatment.

Aspect	Basic Research	Clinical Research	Translational Research
Focus	Discovery	Testing	Application
Subjects	Cells, animals	Humans	Patients and populations
Goal	Knowledge generation	Safety and efficacy testing	Real-world implementation

Examples Of Success In Translational Medicine

1. Insulin for Diabetes Management

- **T0:** Discovery of insulin by Frederick Banting and Charles Best in 1921.
- **T1:** Early clinical trials to test the safety and efficacy of insulin injections.
- **T2:** Large-scale clinical trials confirmed its therapeutic role.
- **T3:** Development of standardized protocols for insulin administration in diabetic care.
- **T4:** Global adoption of insulin therapy, transforming diabetes from a fatal condition to a manageable disease.

2. The mRNA COVID-19 Vaccine

- **T0:** Decades of basic research on mRNA technology and viral immunology.
- **T1:** Preclinical studies showing mRNA's potential to elicit an immune response.
- **T2:** Rapid clinical trials demonstrating safety and efficacy.
- **T3:** Emergency use authorizations enabled large-scale vaccination campaigns.
- **T4:** Ongoing evaluation of vaccine impact on global

COVID-19 morbidity and mortality.

3. Imatinib for Chronic Myeloid Leukemia (CML)

- **T0:** Discovery of the Philadelphia chromosome as a genetic driver of CML.
- **T1:** Development and early testing of Imatinib, a tyrosine kinase inhibitor.
- **T2:** Clinical trials proving its efficacy in achieving remission in CML patients.
- **T3:** Integration into CML treatment guidelines, replacing older therapies.
- **T4:** Improved survival rates for CML patients worldwide.

CHAPTER 2: THE RESEARCH-TO-PATIENT PIPELINE

Translational medicine is often described as a pipeline, moving discoveries from the research lab (bench) to the clinical setting (bedside) and ultimately to public health (population impact).

From Bench To Bedside: Steps In Translating Research

Translating research into patient care involves a systematic and iterative process that ensures safety, efficacy, and practical implementation.

The key steps include:

1. Discovery Phase (Basic Science)

- **Objective:** Uncover biological mechanisms or identify therapeutic targets.
- **Activities:**
    - Conducting laboratory experiments to understand disease processes.
    - Identifying potential drug targets, biomarkers, or pathways.
    - Developing hypotheses about interventions.
- **Example:** Discovery of the role of VEGF (vascular endothelial growth factor) in promoting tumor growth, leading to anti-angiogenesis strategies.

2. Preclinical Development

- **Objective:** Assess the feasibility, safety, and potential

efficacy of a discovery in non-human models.
- **Activities:**
    - Animal studies to evaluate toxicity, dosing, and pharmacokinetics.
    - Refinement of drug formulations or delivery mechanisms.
- **Example:** Testing monoclonal antibodies targeting HER2 in mouse models before human trials.

3. Clinical Trials

- **Objective:** Validate safety and efficacy in humans through phased testing.
- **Phases:**
    - **Phase I:** Focus on safety, dosage, and side effects in a small group of healthy volunteers or patients.
    - **Phase II:** Assess efficacy and optimal dosing in a larger group.
    - **Phase III:** Confirm efficacy, monitor side effects, and compare to standard treatments in a broad population.
- **Example:** Testing the safety and effectiveness of mRNA-based vaccines in large, diverse populations.

4. Regulatory Approval

- **Objective:** Obtain authorization from regulatory agencies such as the FDA, EMA, or other bodies.
- **Activities:**
    - Submitting a comprehensive dossier of preclinical and clinical trial data.
    - Addressing regulatory inquiries and meeting compliance standards.
- **Example:** Gaining FDA approval for CAR-T cell therapy for specific cancers.

5. Implementation in Clinical Practice

- **Objective:** Integrate new therapies or diagnostics into routine healthcare.
- **Activities:**
  - Developing clinical guidelines and educational materials for practitioners.
  - Establishing supply chains and distribution systems.
- **Example:** Training oncologists to use targeted therapies and monitoring systems for personalized cancer care.

6. Post-Market Surveillance

- **Objective:** Monitor real-world effectiveness and long-term safety.
- **Activities:**
  - Conducting Phase IV studies and collecting data from registries.
  - Refining treatment protocols based on feedback.
- **Example:** Long-term safety studies for immunotherapies to identify rare side effects.

Challenges In Bridging The Gap

Despite the structured pipeline, numerous challenges hinder the translation of research into practical applications:

1. Scientific and Technical Challenges

- **Complexity of Biology:** Diseases such as cancer and neurodegenerative disorders involve intricate pathways, making target identification and validation challenging.
- **Preclinical Models:** Animal models may not always

predict human responses accurately.

2. Financial and Resource Constraints

- **High Costs:** The journey from discovery to implementation often requires billions of dollars.
- **Funding Gaps:** Limited funding for translational and early-phase clinical research can delay progress.

3. Regulatory and Ethical Hurdles

- **Regulatory Requirements:** Meeting stringent safety and efficacy criteria can prolong timelines.
- **Ethical Considerations:** Protecting patient rights and ensuring equitable access are ongoing challenges.

4. Collaboration and Communication Barriers

- **Disciplinary Silos:** Poor communication between basic scientists, clinicians, and industry stakeholders can impede progress.
- **Data Sharing:** Proprietary concerns often limit the sharing of data critical to advancing research.

5. Implementation Barriers

- **Healthcare System Readiness:** Integrating new therapies requires training, infrastructure, and changes to clinical workflows.
- **Cost of Care:** Expensive innovations may not be accessible to all patients.

Case Studies Of Breakthrough Innovations

Case Study 1: Crispr-Cas9 Gene Editing

- **Discovery Phase:** Identification of the CRISPR-Cas9 system as a bacterial defense mechanism against viruses.
- **Translation Steps:**
    - Preclinical development demonstrated its potential to edit genes in mammalian cells.
    - Clinical trials focused on treating genetic disorders such as sickle cell anemia and beta-thalassemia.
    - Regulatory pathways ensured compliance with safety standards for human trials.
- **Impact:**
    - Enabled precise gene editing with implications for curing genetic diseases.
    - Paved the way for ethical discussions and policy development in gene editing.

Case Study 2: Human Papillomavirus (Hpv) Vaccine

- **Discovery Phase:** Research linking HPV to cervical cancer led to vaccine development.
- **Translation Steps:**
    - Preclinical testing ensured safety and immunogenicity.

TRANSLATIONAL MEDICINE

- ◦ Large-scale clinical trials demonstrated high efficacy in preventing HPV infections.
- ◦ Regulatory approvals enabled global vaccination programs.
- **Impact:**
  - ◦ Significant reductions in cervical cancer incidence and mortality.
  - ◦ Ongoing campaigns to increase vaccine accessibility in low-income regions.

Case Study 3: Mrna-Based Covid-19 Vaccines

- **Discovery Phase:** Decades of research on mRNA technology provided the foundation.
- **Translation Steps:**
  - ◦ Rapid preclinical and clinical testing during the pandemic accelerated progress.
  - ◦ Emergency use authorizations facilitated early distribution while Phase III trials continued.
- **Impact:**
  - ◦ Saved millions of lives and curbed the spread of COVID-19.
  - ◦ Established a new platform for vaccine development for future pandemics.

CHAPTER 3: ETHICAL CONSIDERATIONS

Ethics plays a pivotal role in translational medicine, ensuring that scientific advancements do not come at the expense of patient rights, safety, and dignity.

Ethical Challenges In Translational Medicine

Translational medicine bridges basic science, clinical research, and patient care, creating unique ethical complexities at each stage of the pipeline.

1. Balancing Innovation and Risk
- **Challenge:** Translational medicine involves introducing novel treatments with limited data, which can expose patients to unforeseen risks.
- **Example:** Early trials of gene-editing technologies like CRISPR raise concerns about unintended genetic mutations.
- **Resolution:** Rigorous preclinical testing, robust risk assessments, and clear communication with participants.

2. Equity and Access
- **Challenge:** Many breakthroughs, such as advanced biologics or personalized therapies, are prohibitively expensive and inaccessible to underserved populations.
- **Example:** CAR-T therapy for cancer is highly effective but remains out of reach for many due to cost.

- **Resolution:** Advocacy for equitable distribution, public funding for innovative treatments, and tiered pricing models.

3. Dual-Use Concerns
- **Challenge:** Some research has potential dual uses, meaning it could benefit society but also be misused.
- **Example:** Gain-of-function research on viruses for vaccine development carries risks of accidental or deliberate misuse.
- **Resolution:** Transparent governance, international oversight, and stringent biosafety protocols.

4. Conflicts of Interest
- **Challenge:** Industry funding for translational research can create conflicts between commercial interests and patient welfare.
- **Example:** Researchers involved in trials of a drug they have financial stakes in may face bias.
- **Resolution:** Full disclosure of conflicts, independent oversight, and peer review processes.

Informed Consent In Clinical Trials

Informed consent is the cornerstone of ethical research, ensuring that participants fully understand the nature of the study and agree to participate voluntarily.

1. Core Principles of Informed Consent
- **Autonomy:** Participants must have the freedom to decide without coercion or undue influence.
- **Comprehension:** Information provided must be clear, comprehensive, and accessible.
- **Disclosure:** All relevant details, including risks, benefits, and alternatives, must be shared.

- **Voluntariness:** Participation must be entirely voluntary, with the option to withdraw at any time.

2. Challenges in Achieving Genuine Consent

- **Scientific Complexity:** Translational studies often involve highly technical information that is difficult for laypersons to understand.
- **Therapeutic Misconception:** Participants may confuse trial participation with receiving established treatments, believing the research is tailored to their benefit.
- **Vulnerable Populations:** Patients with terminal illnesses or limited healthcare access may feel pressured to join experimental trials.

3. Strategies for Enhancing Informed Consent

- **Simplified Language:** Use plain language summaries and visual aids to explain study details.
- **Continuous Consent:** Treat consent as an ongoing dialogue rather than a one-time formality.
- **Independent Advocacy:** Employ patient advocates or ethics boards to guide participants.
- **Tailored Approaches:** Adapt consent processes to the cultural, linguistic, and educational backgrounds of participants.

Balancing Research And Patient Safety

Advancing science while safeguarding patient welfare is a delicate balance that requires adherence to ethical principles and regulatory standards.

1. Rigorous Preclinical Testing
- **Objective:** Minimize risks to humans by thoroughly evaluating safety and efficacy in vitro and in animal models.
- **Example:** Testing COVID-19 vaccines on animal models before human trials ensured safety while accelerating the process under emergency use protocols.

2. Ethical Oversight and Governance
- **Institutional Review Boards (IRBs):** Assess trial protocols for ethical compliance.
- **Data Safety Monitoring Boards (DSMBs):** Monitor ongoing trials to detect and mitigate adverse events.
- **Ethical Frameworks:** Guidelines such as the Declaration of Helsinki and the Belmont Report provide standards for patient safety.

3. Risk-Benefit Analysis
- **Objective:** Ensure that the potential benefits of research outweigh the risks.
- **Application:** For trials involving high-risk interventions like stem cell therapy, researchers must demonstrate robust preclinical evidence to justify human testing.

4. Transparency and Communication
- **Patient Communication:** Keep participants informed of new developments, adverse events, or changes in study design.

- **Public Accountability:** Disclose results, including negative outcomes, to maintain trust in research.

PART II: KEY COMPONENTS AND STAKEHOLDERS

CHAPTER 4: COLLABORATIONS IN TRANSLATIONAL MEDICINE

Collaboration is the foundation of translational medicine, requiring seamless integration among diverse stakeholders to drive research from the laboratory to the clinic.

Role Of Multidisciplinary Teams

Translational medicine involves multiple scientific disciplines and clinical specialties working together toward a common goal: improving patient outcomes.

1. Composition of Multidisciplinary Teams

- **Basic Scientists:** Provide foundational knowledge, develop hypotheses, and conduct laboratory research.
- **Clinicians:** Offer insights into patient needs, identify clinical challenges, and oversee trials.
- **Biostatisticians and Data Scientists:** Analyze data from preclinical and clinical studies to identify trends and validate findings.
- **Regulatory Experts:** Ensure compliance with guidelines from agencies like the FDA or EMA.
- **Ethicists:** Address ethical concerns, including patient consent and risk-benefit analysis.
- **Healthcare Economists:** Assess the cost-effectiveness and accessibility of interventions.

2. Benefits of Multidisciplinary Collaboration

- **Enhanced Problem-Solving:** Diverse expertise fosters

innovative solutions to complex problems.
- **Accelerated Translation:** Integrated efforts streamline the transition from discovery to application.
- **Improved Patient Outcomes:** Collaboration ensures that new therapies align with clinical realities and patient needs.

3. Challenges and Solutions
- **Challenge:** Communication barriers due to varying terminologies and priorities among disciplines.
- **Solution:** Establishing shared goals, using plain language, and fostering mutual respect.
- **Challenge:** Managing conflicts over intellectual property or credit allocation.
- **Solution:** Clear agreements and transparent governance frameworks.

Engaging Patients And Communities In Research

Patient-centered research is a hallmark of modern translational medicine, emphasizing the importance of including patients and communities in the research process.

1. Benefits of Patient and Community Engagement
- **Identifying Unmet Needs:** Patients provide real-world insights into their experiences, helping researchers prioritize impactful projects.
- **Improved Study Design:** Incorporating patient perspectives ensures trials are feasible, relevant, and ethically sound.
- **Enhanced Trust and Participation:** Engaging communities fosters trust, increases trial enrollment, and reduces dropout rates.

2. Methods of Engagement

- **Patient Advisory Boards:** Groups of patients and caregivers provide feedback on research priorities and trial protocols.
- **Community-Based Participatory Research (CBPR):** A collaborative approach involving communities as equal partners in the research process.
- **Focus Groups and Surveys:** Gather qualitative and quantitative data on patient experiences and preferences.

3. Ethical Considerations in Engagement
- **Informed Participation:** Patients must understand their role and rights when engaging in research.
- **Representation and Equity:** Efforts should be made to engage diverse populations, including underserved groups, to ensure equitable access to research benefits.

Partnerships Between Academia, Industry, And Government

Collaboration across sectors is crucial for bridging the research-to-patient gap, leveraging the strengths of academia, industry, and government entities.

1. Academia's Role
- **Core Strengths:** Fundamental research, innovation, and education.
- **Challenges:** Limited funding and resources for large-scale trials.
- **Opportunities:** Partnerships with industry and government can scale promising discoveries into clinical applications.

2. Industry's Role

- **Core Strengths:** Expertise in drug development, manufacturing, and commercialization.
- **Challenges:** Balancing profit motives with public health priorities.
- **Opportunities:** Collaborating with academia for innovation and government for regulatory support.

3. Government's Role

- **Core Strengths:** Funding initiatives (e.g., NIH, Horizon Europe), establishing regulatory frameworks, and ensuring equitable access.
- **Challenges:** Bureaucratic processes can slow innovation.
- **Opportunities:** Public-private partnerships and policies that incentivize innovation.

4. Models of Collaboration

- **Public-Private Partnerships (PPPs):** Combine resources and expertise from public and private sectors.
  - **Example:** The Accelerating COVID-19 Therapeutic Interventions and Vaccines (ACTIV) initiative brought together NIH, industry, and nonprofits to speed up COVID-19 research.
- **Academic-Industry Alliances:** Collaborations like the Broad Institute's partnerships with biotech companies accelerate genomic research applications.
- **Regulatory Science Collaborations:** FDA's Critical Path Initiative engages academia and industry to improve drug development pathways.

CHAPTER 5: ROLE OF TECHNOLOGY AND INNOVATION

Technological advancements and innovation are revolutionizing translational medicine, enabling faster, more precise, and more effective pathways from research to patient care.

Big Data And Artificial Intelligence In Translational Research

1. The Role of Big Data in Translational Medicine

Big data refers to the vast amounts of structured and unstructured data generated from various sources, including clinical trials, electronic health records (EHRs), genomics, and wearable devices. Translational research leverages this data to identify patterns, generate hypotheses, and personalize treatments.

- **Data Sources:**
    - Clinical trial databases.
    - Biobanks and genomic datasets.
    - Real-world evidence from EHRs and patient registries.
    - Sensor and wearable data (e.g., fitness trackers, implantable devices).
- **Applications in Translational Medicine:**
    - **Identifying Biomarkers:** Analysis of genomic and proteomic data to discover disease-specific biomarkers.
    - **Drug Repurposing:** Mining existing datasets

to identify new therapeutic uses for approved drugs.
- **Predicting Treatment Outcomes:** Using patient data to forecast responses to therapies.

2. Artificial Intelligence In Translational Medicine

AI, particularly machine learning and deep learning, has become a cornerstone in processing and interpreting big data in translational medicine.

- **Applications of AI:**
  - **Diagnostics:** AI algorithms analyze imaging data (e.g., CT scans, MRIs) for early disease detection.
  - **Drug Discovery:** Machine learning identifies potential drug candidates and predicts their efficacy.
  - **Clinical Trial Optimization:** AI identifies eligible participants, predicts trial outcomes, and reduces dropout rates.
- **Case Study:**
  - **AlphaFold:** An AI tool developed by DeepMind has revolutionized protein structure prediction, enabling breakthroughs in drug discovery and understanding of diseases at the molecular level.

Challenges And Ethical Considerations:

- **Data Privacy:** Ensuring patient confidentiality while sharing data for research purposes.
- **Bias in AI Models:** Addressing biases arising from

underrepresented populations in datasets.
- **Integration:** Overcoming technical and organizational barriers to integrating big data into clinical workflows.

Precision Medicine And Genomics Applications

Precision medicine tailors treatment to individual variability in genes, environment, and lifestyle. Genomics, a cornerstone of precision medicine, is transforming translational research by enabling targeted therapies and personalized healthcare.

1. Precision Medicine in Translational Research

- **Concept:** Treatments are designed based on the molecular profile of an individual rather than a one-size-fits-all approach.
- **Impact:** Improves efficacy, reduces adverse effects, and enhances patient outcomes.
- **Examples of Precision Medicine Applications:**
    - **Oncology:** Targeted therapies like trastuzumab for HER2-positive breast cancer and osimertinib for EGFR-mutant lung cancer.
    - **Cardiology:** Pharmacogenomics to guide anticoagulant therapy (e.g., warfarin dosing based on genetic variants).

2. Genomics in Translational Medicine

- **Genome-Wide Association Studies (GWAS):** Identify genetic variations linked to diseases, aiding in biomarker discovery.
- **CRISPR-Cas9 Technology:** Allows precise editing of genetic material, paving the way for gene therapies.
- **Case Study:**
    - **Sickle Cell Disease Gene Therapy:**

Researchers used CRISPR to edit the gene responsible for sickle cell disease, achieving promising results in early trials.

3. Challenges and Limitations:
- **Cost:** High costs of genomic testing and targeted therapies can limit accessibility.
- **Data Interpretation:** Requires specialized expertise to analyze complex genomic data.
- **Ethical Concerns:** Issues related to genetic editing, data privacy, and equitable access.

Tools For Monitoring And Evaluating Outcomes

The ability to monitor and evaluate the outcomes of translational research is crucial for assessing the impact of interventions, ensuring patient safety, and refining therapeutic strategies.

1. Digital Health Technologies
- **Wearable Devices:**
  - Monitor vital signs, physical activity, and disease symptoms in real time.
  - Examples: Continuous glucose monitors for diabetes, wearable ECG devices for arrhythmias.
- **Remote Patient Monitoring (RPM):**
  - Enables data collection from patients in their natural environments, reducing the need for frequent clinic visits.
  - Example: Telehealth platforms for chronic disease management.

2. Advanced Imaging Techniques
- **Functional MRI (fMRI):** Tracks real-time changes in brain activity, aiding in neurology and psychiatry

research.
- **PET-CT Scans:** Evaluate metabolic activity in tissues, crucial for cancer diagnosis and monitoring.

3. Biomarker-Based Monitoring
- **Definition:** Biological indicators, such as proteins or metabolites, that reflect disease state or treatment response.
- **Applications:**
  - Monitor cancer progression using circulating tumor DNA (ctDNA).
  - Evaluate drug toxicity through liver and kidney function biomarkers.

4. AI-Driven Outcome Analysis
- AI tools analyze patient data to assess treatment effectiveness and predict long-term outcomes.
  - Example: AI-powered predictive models for assessing risks of cardiovascular events after interventions.

5. Registries and Real-World Evidence (RWE):
- Patient registries collect longitudinal data on treatments and outcomes, providing real-world insights beyond clinical trials.
- RWE supports post-market surveillance and ongoing evaluation of therapeutic interventions.

CHAPTER 6: REGULATORY PATHWAYS

The regulatory process is a crucial component of translational medicine, ensuring that new therapies, treatments, and medical technologies are both safe and effective before they reach patients.

Regulatory agencies, most notably the U.S. Food and Drug Administration (FDA) and the European Medicines Agency (EMA), play a pivotal role in overseeing the approval of drugs, biologics, and devices.

Understanding The Role Of The Fda And Ema

1. The U.S. Food and Drug Administration (FDA)

The FDA is the regulatory authority responsible for approving drugs, biologics, medical devices, and other healthcare products in the United States.

It operates under the U.S. Department of Health and Human Services and is tasked with protecting public health by ensuring that products meet rigorous standards for safety, efficacy, and quality.

- **Primary Functions of the FDA:**
    - **Drug Approval:** The FDA evaluates and approves new drugs, ensuring they are safe and effective for their intended use.
    - **Biologics Regulation:** It oversees biologics, including vaccines, blood products, gene therapies, and cell therapies.

- **Medical Device Regulation:** The FDA also regulates medical devices ranging from simple bandages to complex surgical instruments.
- **Food Safety:** Ensures the safety of food products, supplements, and cosmetics.
- **Post-Market Surveillance:** Once products are approved, the FDA monitors their ongoing safety and effectiveness through post-market studies and adverse event reporting systems.

- **FDA Drug Approval Process:**
  - **Preclinical Testing:** Before clinical trials, drugs undergo preclinical testing in laboratories and animal models.
  - **Clinical Trials (Phase I-III):** Drugs move through human clinical trials to evaluate their safety, dosage, effectiveness, and side effects.
  - **New Drug Application (NDA):** Following successful clinical trials, a company submits an NDA to the FDA, which includes all data on the drug's safety, efficacy, and manufacturing process.
  - **FDA Review:** The FDA reviews the NDA, often with advisory committees, to decide whether the drug should be approved for market use.

2. The European Medicines Agency (Ema)

The EMA is the European Union's (EU) counterpart to the FDA, responsible for the evaluation and supervision of medicinal products in the EU. It harmonizes the drug approval process across the 27 member states, ensuring that treatments meet safety standards and are accessible to EU patients.

- **Primary Functions of the EMA:**
  - **Centralized Authorization Procedure:** The EMA oversees a single application process for marketing approval in all EU member states.
  - **Scientific Evaluation:** The agency assesses medicinal products, including drugs, vaccines, and advanced therapies (e.g., gene therapies).
  - **Pharmacovigilance:** The EMA monitors the safety of authorized medicines through adverse event reporting and risk management.
  - **Advisory Committees:** Like the FDA, the EMA uses advisory committees to provide expert reviews of drug applications and clinical trial data.
- **EMA Drug Approval Process:**
  - **Preclinical Studies:** Like the FDA, preclinical studies are conducted before human testing.
  - **Clinical Trials (Phases I-III):** Drugs undergo clinical trials in human participants to evaluate their safety and efficacy.
  - **Marketing Authorization Application (MAA):** The MAA is submitted to the EMA, detailing the product's development and clinical trial results.
  - **EMA Evaluation:** The agency evaluates the application with input from its scientific committees, such as the Committee for Medicinal Products for Human Use (CHMP), and then makes a recommendation for approval.

Drug Development And Approval Processes

1. Stages of Drug Development

Drug development is a lengthy and complex process that can take several years to complete. The stages of development include:

- **Discovery and Preclinical Research:**
  The initial stage focuses on identifying potential drug candidates through basic research, followed by laboratory testing and animal studies. Preclinical research helps establish the drug's pharmacodynamics, pharmacokinetics, and toxicity profile.

- **Clinical Trials:**
  Once a promising drug is identified, clinical trials are conducted in humans to evaluate its safety and effectiveness. Clinical trials are divided into three phases:
    - **Phase I:** Focuses on safety, dosing, and side effects in a small group of healthy volunteers.
    - **Phase II:** Expands the trial to patients with the disease of interest, testing the drug's efficacy and safety at different doses.
    - **Phase III:** Large-scale trials compare the new drug to existing treatments, testing its long-term safety, effectiveness, and rare side effects.

- **Regulatory Submission and Review:**
  Following the completion of clinical trials, a company submits a New Drug Application (NDA) or Marketing Authorization Application (MAA) to the relevant regulatory agency (FDA or EMA). The application includes all clinical trial data, manufacturing processes, and labeling information.

- **Approval and Post-Market Surveillance:**
  After review, the regulatory agency approves the drug for use. However, post-market surveillance continues to monitor for any adverse effects or issues that may arise during real-world use.

2. Challenges In Drug Development And Approval:

- **High Costs and Time:** Drug development is expensive, with costs often exceeding $1 billion and timelines stretching over 10-15 years.
- **Failure Rates:** Many drug candidates fail at various stages, especially in clinical trials, due to safety concerns or lack of efficacy.
- **Regulatory Hurdles:** Navigating complex regulatory processes can be challenging, especially for novel therapies like biologics, gene therapies, and rare disease treatments.

Fast-Track And Breakthrough Designations

In an effort to expedite the development of therapies for serious conditions, the FDA and EMA have established special regulatory designations, such as the **Fast-Track** and **Breakthrough Therapy Designations**.

1. Fast-Track Designation (Fda)

The **Fast-Track** designation is granted to drugs that treat serious conditions and fill an unmet medical need. It is designed to speed up the development and review process for these treatments.

- **Criteria for Fast-Track Designation:**
    - The drug must treat a serious condition or disease.
    - There must be no adequate treatment available, or the new drug must offer a significant benefit over existing treatments.
    - The FDA accelerates interactions with sponsors, including more frequent meetings and guidance on trial designs.
- **Benefits:**
    - Rolling review: The FDA may review portions of the NDA as they are completed, rather than waiting for all data to be submitted.
    - Priority review: The FDA expedites the review process, reducing the standard review time.
- **Example:**
    - **Sovaldi (sofosbuvir):** A drug for hepatitis C, received fast-track designation and was approved rapidly due to its ability to cure hepatitis C in a short time with fewer side

effects.

2. Breakthrough Therapy Designation (Fda)

The **Breakthrough Therapy Designation** is designed for drugs that show preliminary evidence of substantial improvement over existing treatments for serious conditions. It offers a more comprehensive level of support compared to Fast-Track.

- **Criteria for Breakthrough Therapy Designation:**
  - The drug must treat a serious condition.
  - Preliminary clinical evidence must indicate that the drug shows substantial improvement on at least one clinically significant endpoint.
- **Benefits:**
  - Intensive guidance on clinical trial design and additional meetings with FDA staff.
  - Eligibility for accelerated approval and rolling reviews.
- **Example:**
  - **Kymriah (tisagenlecleucel):** A gene therapy for certain types of leukemia, received Breakthrough Therapy Designation for its significant impact on patient survival.

3. Accelerated Approval Pathway (Ema And Fda)

Both the FDA and EMA have accelerated approval pathways, designed to bring treatments to market faster for serious diseases. These pathways allow for drugs to be approved based on surrogate endpoints (indicators that predict clinical benefit but are not directly measured by the outcome of interest) rather than definitive clinical evidence.

- **Example:**
    - **Keytruda (pembrolizumab):** A checkpoint inhibitor used in various cancers, was granted accelerated approval for non-small cell lung cancer based on early-stage evidence.

CHAPTER 7: BRIDGING THE RESEARCH FUNDING GAP

Research in translational medicine—turning laboratory discoveries into practical treatments for patients—requires substantial funding at every stage of development.

However, securing adequate financial resources can be one of the most significant challenges researchers face, as the pathway from bench to bedside is often lengthy, complex, and costly.

Funding Challenges In Translational Medicine

1. High Costs and Long Timelines

One of the most prominent challenges in translational research is the high cost involved. Moving from basic research (T0) to clinical trials (T1-T3) and eventually to widespread clinical application (T4) requires significant financial investment. These expenses include:

- **Preclinical Development:** The early stages of drug discovery involve laboratory research, animal testing, and optimization of compounds or therapies, which require expensive equipment, reagents, and laboratory staff.
- **Clinical Trials:** Human trials are notoriously costly, particularly Phase III trials, which often involve thousands of patients. The need for extensive monitoring, regulatory compliance, data collection, and long-term follow-up adds to the expense.
- **Regulatory Approval:** Navigating the regulatory

process, including compiling and submitting comprehensive data to regulatory agencies like the FDA and EMA, requires significant resources for legal, clinical, and operational costs.

- **Commercialization and Distribution:** After approval, scaling production, establishing distribution channels, and post-market surveillance can incur further costs, making translational medicine a highly resource-intensive process.

Because of these high costs, researchers and companies may face difficulties in securing long-term funding, especially when they are unsure whether their investments will yield successful, marketable results.

2. Risk of Failure

Translational research, by nature, carries high risks. The vast majority of drug candidates fail at various stages of development due to safety issues, lack of efficacy, or unforeseen side effects. As a result, investors may be hesitant to provide funding for initiatives that have uncertain outcomes, leading to a funding gap in the later stages of research, where financial support is most needed.

Many translational medicine projects struggle to obtain consistent funding as they move into costly human trials, where risk of failure is higher, and results are often difficult to predict. As such, the uncertainty surrounding these ventures poses a barrier to researchers seeking consistent financial backing.

3. Limited Public Funding

Public funding, from sources such as government agencies, foundations, and charitable organizations, is essential for many translational research projects. However, the availability of these funds is often limited due to budgetary constraints, political priorities, and competition from other healthcare and research sectors.

Government agencies, including the U.S. National Institutes of Health (NIH) and the European Commission, provide substantial funding for biomedical research, but the focus is often on basic science rather than translational research. This leaves a gap in funding that may not be filled by private investors due to the aforementioned risks and costs.

Innovative Financing Models And Grant Opportunities

As traditional funding sources alone may not suffice to meet the financial needs of translational research, new and innovative financing models are emerging to help bridge the funding gap.

These models aim to attract investments and accelerate the development of new therapies. Here are several approaches gaining momentum in the field:

1. Public-Private Partnerships (Ppps)

Public-private partnerships (PPPs) bring together government funding and private sector investment to support translational research.

These collaborations leverage the strengths of both sectors —government funding can provide long-term support and regulatory expertise, while private companies can provide the innovation, expertise in commercialization, and additional financial backing needed to bring therapies to market.

- **Example:** The **Coalition for Epidemic Preparedness Innovations (CEPI)** is a partnership that helps fund the development of vaccines for emerging infectious diseases. CEPI brings together governments, philanthropic organizations, and private companies to accelerate the development of vaccines that can be produced quickly in response to global health crises.

2. Venture Capital And Angel Investors

Venture capital (VC) firms and angel investors are increasingly stepping in to provide funding for translational medicine projects, especially those focused on early-stage innovations.

These investors are often willing to take on higher risks in exchange for potential high returns if the therapy succeeds.

- **Example: Theranos**, despite its later controversies, initially secured large investments from venture capitalists eager to capitalize on innovative healthcare technology. Successful companies like **Moderna** and **BioNTech**, which developed mRNA vaccines for COVID-19, also attracted significant VC investments early on, enabling them to progress from the research stage to clinical trials.

3. Crowdfunding And Social Impact Investment

Crowdfunding has emerged as a popular model for securing research funding, especially for smaller, early-stage translational medicine projects that may not attract traditional venture capital or large public grants. Platforms like **GoFundMe**, **Indiegogo**, and specialized medical *crowdfunding platforms* such as **Experiment.com** allow researchers to present their work to the general public, raising small amounts of money from large numbers of individual donors.

Social impact investing, which focuses on generating measurable social or environmental impacts alongside financial returns, has also gained traction. Impact investors seek to fund projects that promise not only a return on investment but also the potential to create meaningful social or health improvements.

- **Example: Cancer Research UK** raised significant funds through crowdfunding campaigns for specific research initiatives, allowing the public to directly contribute to the development of potential life-saving treatments.

4. Innovative Government Grants And Initiatives

Governments and international organizations have established targeted funding initiatives to support translational medicine.

These grants typically focus on specific therapeutic areas or public health challenges, such as cancer, rare diseases, or infectious diseases.

- **Example:** The **U.S. Department of Defense (DoD)** and **Biomedical Advanced Research and Development Authority (BARDA)** have special funding programs that focus on the development of medical countermeasures for bioterrorism, pandemics, and other public health emergencies.
- **Example:** The **Innovative Medicines Initiative (IMI)**, a European Commission initiative, funds collaborative projects that address unmet medical needs and support the development of new medicines, focusing on innovative areas such as antibiotics, immunotherapies, and rare diseases.

Global Perspectives On Research Funding

Translational research funding varies across countries and regions, with different systems in place to foster innovation, manage risks, and prioritize research. Here are key perspectives on how research funding is approached globally:

1. United States: A Leader In Biomedical Innovation

The United States is a global leader in biomedical research funding, driven by government agencies such as the NIH, as well as private sector investments and venture capital. U.S. funding supports a broad spectrum of translational research, from basic science to clinical trials and commercialization.

- **Challenges:** Despite the abundant funding opportunities, the U.S. faces challenges in ensuring that funding is allocated to the most innovative and high-priority projects. Moreover, there are concerns regarding equitable access to funding for underserved populations and emerging researchers.

2. European Union: Coordinated Funding Across Member States

The European Union has a centralized system for translational research funding, with programs like **Horizon Europe** supporting innovation and collaboration between countries. Europe encourages cross-border partnerships to tackle diseases that affect the entire continent, such as cancer, diabetes, and neurodegenerative disorders.

- **Challenges:** The funding landscape in the EU is often fragmented, as each member state has its own national funding schemes. Researchers may face difficulties navigating these diverse systems, and competition for limited resources can be intense.

3. Low- And Middle-Income Countries: Addressing Global Health Challenges

In many low- and middle-income countries (LMICs), research funding for translational medicine is limited, which impacts efforts to develop treatments for diseases that disproportionately affect these populations. International organizations, such as the **World Health Organization (WHO)** and **Gavi**, are stepping in to support research focused on diseases like malaria, tuberculosis, and neglected tropical diseases.

- **Challenges:** LMICs face significant barriers to conducting translational research, including inadequate infrastructure, lack of trained researchers, and limited access to funding. Addressing these challenges requires innovative funding models, such as partnerships between international organizations, governments, and the private sector.

CHAPTER 8: OVERCOMING BARRIERS IN IMPLEMENTATION

Translational medicine aims to transform scientific discoveries from the laboratory into tangible treatments that benefit patients. However, the journey from research to clinical application is often riddled with significant barriers that hinder the successful implementation of promising innovations.

These challenges can stem from technical, regulatory, economic, and cultural factors that create bottlenecks in the process.

Translational Research Bottlenecks

The path from research to patient care is a multi-step process, and each phase presents its own set of challenges.

Identifying and understanding *these bottlenecks* is essential for developing effective strategies to overcome them.

1. Scientific and Technical Barriers

- **Preclinical to Clinical Transition:** One of the most significant bottlenecks in translational medicine is the transition from preclinical (bench) research to human clinical trials. While preclinical studies may show promising results in animal models, translating these findings to human populations is often difficult due to differences in biology, drug metabolism, and disease pathophysiology. Not all treatments that appear effective in animals or laboratory settings work in humans.
- **Lack of Validated Biomarkers:** In many cases, there is

a lack of reliable biomarkers that can predict patient responses to treatments. Without robust biomarkers, it becomes challenging to identify which patients are most likely to benefit from a specific intervention, leading to ineffective clinical trials and wasted resources.

- **Inadequate Models:** The existing animal models or cell-based systems often do not fully capture the complexities of human disease, which limits the applicability of results. For example, animal models may not reflect the human immune system's complexity, resulting in treatments that show promise in animals but fail in human trials.

2. Regulatory Hurdles

- **Lengthy Approval Processes:** Regulatory agencies, such as the **FDA** (U.S. Food and Drug Administration) and **EMA** (European Medicines Agency), have rigorous processes for evaluating new drugs and treatments. These processes are essential for patient safety but can be time-consuming and expensive, which often delays the implementation of novel therapies.
- **Uncertainty in Approval:** The approval of new treatments often involves unpredictable outcomes. Even well-designed clinical trials may fail to demonstrate sufficient evidence to secure regulatory approval, leading to frustration among researchers and investors and slowing the translation of research into practice.
- **Fragmentation of Regulatory Systems:** The regulatory landscape for translational research can vary significantly between countries and regions, creating confusion and delays in implementing new treatments globally. The lack of harmonization

between regulatory authorities can create additional hurdles for researchers seeking to bring their innovations to multiple markets.

3. Financial Barriers

- **Insufficient Funding:** As discussed in Chapter 7, obtaining adequate funding for translational medicine remains one of the most critical challenges. Many early-stage translational projects struggle to secure financing, particularly during clinical trial stages where costs escalate significantly. Moreover, many funding agencies prioritize basic science research over translational efforts, further exacerbating this challenge.
- **High Costs of Clinical Trials:** Clinical trials, particularly those in later stages (Phase II and III), can require significant financial resources. Small and medium-sized enterprises (SMEs) and academic researchers may struggle to obtain the necessary funds to move their projects through the regulatory process. This financial burden may discourage innovation or delay the development of life-saving therapies.

4. Market Access And Commercialization

- **Uncertain Market Demand:** Even when new treatments pass clinical trials and regulatory approval, there may be uncertainties surrounding the market demand for these therapies. If a new drug is costly or if the patient population is too small, companies may be hesitant to commercialize the product.
- **Barriers to Distribution:** Issues such as intellectual property rights, patent protections, and international trade regulations can complicate the distribution

of new medical innovations. Access to essential medications may be limited by patents, pricing negotiations, and market monopolies, particularly in low-income countries or emerging markets.

Strategies For Accelerating Implementation

To overcome these bottlenecks and accelerate the implementation of translational research, multiple strategies can be employed. These approaches focus on enhancing collaboration, improving regulatory processes, fostering innovation, and streamlining clinical development.

1. Streamlining Regulatory Processes

- **Regulatory Science Innovation:** Regulatory agencies are increasingly adopting modern tools such as **adaptive clinical trial designs** and **real-time monitoring of clinical trial data**. These innovations allow for more flexible and faster approval processes, particularly for urgent health crises or life-threatening conditions.
- **Early Engagement with Regulators:** Researchers and developers can benefit from early consultation with regulatory agencies, which helps them understand the regulatory landscape and anticipate potential roadblocks. Early regulatory engagement can lead to more efficient trials and smoother approval processes.
- **Global Regulatory Harmonization:** Efforts to harmonize regulations across different countries and regions—such as through the **International Council for Harmonisation (ICH)**—can reduce regulatory burden and expedite the global dissemination of new treatments. Global regulatory partnerships can help align standards and facilitate faster approval across multiple markets.

2. Enhancing Collaboration Between Stakeholders

- **Public-Private Partnerships (PPPs):** Collaborative initiatives between public research institutions, private companies, and government agencies can help overcome funding and resource challenges. PPPs pool resources, share risks, and accelerate the development of new treatments. These collaborations can also help streamline the regulatory process by aligning industry standards with regulatory requirements.
- **Cross-Disciplinary Collaborations:** The involvement of multidisciplinary teams, including researchers, clinicians, engineers, and bioinformaticians, is essential to bridging the gap between basic research and clinical practice. By fostering collaboration between diverse fields, researchers can leverage different perspectives and expertise to address complex challenges in translational medicine.
- **Patient and Community Involvement:** Engaging patients and the wider community in the research process not only improves the relevance of the research but also helps accelerate its adoption. Involving patients in early-stage clinical trials, soliciting their feedback on potential therapies, and educating them about the value of clinical research can lead to increased participation and support.

3. Leveraging Technology And Data

- **Big Data and Artificial Intelligence (AI):** Advanced data analytics tools and AI can accelerate the development of new therapies by identifying patterns and predicting patient outcomes. These tools can be used to analyze large datasets from clinical trials, helping to identify biomarkers, predict adverse reactions, and streamline clinical trial designs.

- **Precision Medicine:** Integrating genomics, proteomics, and other omics technologies into clinical trials enables a more personalized approach to treatment development. Precision medicine allows for the identification of patient subgroups that are most likely to benefit from specific therapies, thus improving the efficiency of clinical trials and treatment effectiveness.

4. Alternative Models Of Clinical Trials

- **Adaptive Clinical Trials:** Adaptive trials allow for modifications to the trial design based on interim data, enabling faster and more efficient decision-making. For example, the **Platform Trials** design, which tests multiple interventions in the same patient population, can provide faster insights into the efficacy of new treatments and avoid unnecessary trial delays.
- **Real-World Evidence (RWE):** Increasingly, researchers are using real-world data (such as electronic health records and patient registries) to supplement traditional clinical trials. RWE can help identify patient populations that are most likely to benefit from a treatment and assess its long-term safety and effectiveness.

Cultural And Institutional Resistance

Despite the availability of strategies to address technical and financial barriers, cultural and institutional resistance remains a significant challenge in the implementation of translational research.

1. Resistance to Change

Healthcare institutions and the medical community, in general, can be resistant to adopting new therapies, particularly when these innovations challenge established practices. This resistance may be due to concerns about patient safety, the perceived complexity of new treatments, or simply inertia within healthcare organizations.

Addressing these concerns requires:

- **Education and Awareness:** Researchers and institutions must invest in educating healthcare providers about the benefits of new treatments and technologies, as well as their potential impact on patient outcomes.
- **Building Trust with Stakeholders:** Ensuring that new treatments are safe, effective, and well-tested through rigorous clinical trials is essential to overcoming skepticism. Building trust among healthcare providers, regulatory bodies, and patients is critical for fostering the widespread adoption of new therapies.

2. Institutional Silos And Bureaucracy

Many healthcare and research institutions operate in silos, making it difficult for different departments or disciplines to collaborate. Institutional bureaucracy, rigid hierarchies, and poor communication can slow down the implementation of translational research.

To overcome these barriers:

- **Creating a Collaborative Culture:** Institutions can encourage interdisciplinary collaboration by breaking down silos and promoting team-based approaches to research. Fostering a culture of innovation, open communication, and mutual respect can help overcome institutional barriers to implementation.
- **Flexible Organizational Structures:** Research institutions and hospitals that embrace flexible

organizational structures are better positioned to adapt to new research findings and implement innovative treatments. Encouraging cross-departmental cooperation and creating platforms for knowledge sharing can accelerate the translation of research into practice.

CHAPTER 9: DATA MANAGEMENT AND SHARING

In translational medicine, the successful translation of research from the laboratory to clinical applications hinges on the efficient and responsible management of data. Research data provides the foundation for developing new therapies, understanding disease mechanisms, and improving patient outcomes.

As translational research becomes increasingly data-driven, the importance of robust data management practices and effective data sharing strategies has never been greater.

Importance Of Data Transparency

Data transparency is a critical aspect of translational research. Open access to research data and the ability to verify results ensures the reproducibility, credibility, and reliability of scientific findings.

Transparent data management practices enhance the integrity of research and foster trust among the scientific community, clinicians, and patients. Data transparency also facilitates collaboration, as shared data can inspire further studies, improve the efficiency of research, and reduce duplication of effort.

1. Enhancing Reproducibility

One of the key reasons for promoting data transparency in translational medicine is to support the reproducibility of research findings.

Reproducibility is a cornerstone of scientific progress, and when research data is shared openly, it allows other scientists to independently verify results, build upon them, or identify inconsistencies.

Lack of data transparency, on the other hand, can lead to irreproducible findings, wasting time and resources, and potentially delaying the introduction of new treatments.

2. Promoting Collaboration

Data transparency also encourages collaboration among researchers, clinicians, and other stakeholders in translational medicine.

By sharing data, researchers can pool resources, combine datasets, and tackle complex scientific questions together.

Collaboration can lead to faster breakthroughs, as different experts contribute their knowledge and skills to analyzing and interpreting data.

3. Accelerating Innovation

With transparent data, the scientific community can more easily identify gaps in knowledge and areas for improvement. Researchers can identify existing datasets that can be used to test new hypotheses, validate experimental treatments, or explore new applications for existing therapies. Open data access accelerates the discovery process, reducing the time it takes to bring innovations from the lab to the clinic.

Navigating Data Privacy And Security

While data transparency is essential, it must be balanced with stringent data privacy and security measures. In translational medicine, particularly in clinical research, much of the data collected involves personal health information (PHI) or sensitive patient data. Protecting patient privacy is paramount, and failure to maintain confidentiality can lead to serious legal and ethical issues.

Researchers must navigate complex regulations governing data privacy and security to ensure that their practices comply with legal standards and safeguard the interests of patients.

1. Regulatory Compliance

- **Health Insurance Portability and Accountability Act (HIPAA):** In the U.S., researchers must comply with HIPAA regulations to protect patient privacy. HIPAA sets national standards for the protection of PHI, ensuring that any data that could identify a patient is handled securely. Researchers must be diligent in removing personally identifiable information (PII) from datasets when sharing them or making them publicly accessible.

- **General Data Protection Regulation (GDPR):** In Europe, the GDPR is one of the most important legal frameworks for data protection. It imposes strict rules on how personal data should be collected, processed, and stored, including specific requirements for obtaining informed consent, limiting access to data, and ensuring data is used solely for the purposes intended. GDPR compliance is critical for researchers handling patient data, as non-compliance can result in heavy fines and loss of trust.

- **Institutional Review Boards (IRBs) and Ethics Committees:** Ethical review bodies, such as IRBs, play an essential role in ensuring that research data is collected, stored, and shared in a manner that protects patient privacy. Before conducting research that involves personal data, researchers must obtain approval from these bodies, ensuring that patient rights and safety are prioritized.

2. Anonymization And De-Identification

To protect patient privacy, researchers must anonymize or de-identify data before sharing it with other researchers or the public.

Anonymization involves removing all identifiers (e.g., names, addresses, phone numbers) from the data, making it impossible to trace back to an individual. De-identification may involve removing or encoding certain variables (e.g., birth dates, medical record numbers) that could potentially identify a person.

While anonymization and de-identification are critical for privacy protection, they can also limit the ability to follow up with patients or link data to individual clinical outcomes in some cases. Striking a balance between patient privacy and research utility is a challenge that researchers must carefully navigate.

3. Data Security Measures

Protecting sensitive data requires robust security measures to prevent unauthorized access, data breaches, and cyberattacks.

Researchers must ensure that data storage and transmission systems are secure, using encryption technologies, secure cloud storage, and other cybersecurity practices to protect data integrity.

- **Data Encryption:** Encryption is essential for ensuring that data is unreadable by unauthorized parties, both in transit (when data is being transferred over networks) and at rest (when data is stored in databases or cloud systems).

- **Access Control and Auditing:** Only authorized personnel should have access to sensitive data, and their actions should be tracked through an auditing system. Implementing role-based access control (RBAC) ensures that researchers only have access to the data necessary for their work.
- **Regular Security Assessments:** Regular cybersecurity assessments, including vulnerability testing and penetration testing, can help identify potential weaknesses in data management systems and prevent security breaches.

Open Science And Collaborative Platforms

Open science is an evolving movement aimed at making scientific research and data more accessible, transparent, and collaborative.

In the context of translational medicine, open science and collaborative platforms are essential tools for accelerating the discovery and implementation of new therapies.

These platforms enable researchers to share data, results, methodologies, and resources with the broader scientific community, improving the efficiency of research and speeding up the process of translating discoveries into clinical practice.

1. Open Data Repositories

Open data repositories allow researchers to share datasets with the global scientific community. These platforms are often hosted by universities, research institutions, or government agencies, and they enable researchers to access and contribute data related to specific diseases, treatments, or clinical trials.

By providing public access to datasets, open repositories promote transparency, reproducibility, and collaboration.

Well-known platforms include:

- **GenBank:** A repository for genetic sequence data, allowing researchers to share and access genomic information.
- **The Cancer Genome Atlas (TCGA):** A comprehensive resource of genomic, transcriptomic, and epigenomic data for cancer research.
- **ClinicalTrials.gov:** A database of clinical trial results that provides transparency about the progress of ongoing and completed studies.

2. Collaborative Platforms And Networks

Collaborative platforms and networks facilitate communication, collaboration, and data-sharing among researchers from diverse institutions and disciplines. These platforms often focus on specific disease areas, treatment modalities, or clinical challenges, fostering collaboration among researchers, clinicians, and even patients. Examples of such platforms include:

- **ResearchGate:** A professional network for researchers where they can share papers, results, and data, as well as connect with other scientists.
- **Open Science Framework (OSF):** A platform for researchers to share data, protocols, and findings, enabling open collaboration across various stages of the research process.
- **Shared platforms in drug discovery:** Platforms like **Open Drug Discovery Platform (ODDP)** provide access to molecular data and computational tools that allow researchers to collaborate on drug development projects.

3. Advantages Of Open Science In Translational Medicine

- **Faster Innovation:** By making data and findings accessible to a wider audience, open science accelerates the pace of innovation. Researchers from different institutions can combine their expertise and resources to solve complex problems, ultimately leading to faster discoveries and the development of new treatments.
- **Increased Public Engagement:** Open science fosters greater engagement with the public, including patients and advocacy groups. Patients can access research data, follow the progress of clinical trials, and participate in studies. Greater transparency fosters trust and confidence in the research process.
- **Improved Reproducibility and Validation:** Open access to research data allows other researchers to validate results, replicate experiments, and test new hypotheses. This reduces the likelihood of false positives and ensures that only the most robust findings are translated into clinical applications.

CHAPTER 10: TRANSLATIONAL MEDICINE IN ONCOLOGY

Translational medicine has significantly impacted oncology, transforming the landscape of cancer treatment and offering hope for patients with previously difficult-to-treat cancers.

Translational medicine bridges the gap between laboratory discoveries and clinical applications, ensuring that innovations in cancer research move swiftly from the bench to the bedside.

Examples Of Cancer Therapies From Research To Practice

In oncology, translational medicine has paved the way for several groundbreaking therapies that were once confined to the laboratory but have since become integral to clinical practice. These therapies include:

1. Targeted Therapies

Targeted therapies represent a paradigm shift in cancer treatment, as they focus on specific molecular targets involved in cancer cell growth and survival. Unlike traditional chemotherapy, which indiscriminately targets fast-dividing cells, targeted therapies aim to interfere with specific proteins or genes that contribute to cancer's development and progression.

- **Example: Trastuzumab (Herceptin)** is a monoclonal antibody targeted against the HER2/neu receptor, overexpressed in some types of breast cancer. The development of trastuzumab began with the identification of HER2 as a driver of breast cancer growth. The translation of this discovery into clinical therapy demonstrated that blocking HER2 with trastuzumab significantly improves patient outcomes in HER2-positive breast cancer.

- **Example: Imatinib (Gleevec)**, a tyrosine kinase inhibitor, targets the BCR-ABL fusion gene present in chronic myelogenous leukemia (CML). Its development was based on research into the molecular mechanisms of CML, particularly the discovery of the BCR-ABL gene fusion. Imatinib revolutionized the treatment of CML by specifically targeting the abnormal protein produced by this fusion gene, leading to durable responses in many patients.

2. Immunotherapy

*Immunotherapy h*as emerged as one of the most promising areas of oncology research. It harnesses the power of the immune system to recognize and attack cancer cells. By targeting immune checkpoints, enhancing the body's immune response, or modifying immune cells, immunotherapies have shown remarkable effectiveness in treating certain cancers, particularly those resistant to traditional treatments.

3. CAR-T Cell Therapy

Chimeric Antigen Receptor T-cell (CAR-T) therapy is one of the most revolutionary breakthroughs in cancer immunotherapy.

This approach involves genetically modifying a patient's own T cells to express receptors that specifically recognize and bind to tumor antigens, thereby enhancing the immune system's ability to target and destroy cancer cells. CAR-T cell therapy has demonstrated exceptional success in the treatment of hematologic cancers, particularly certain types of leukemia and lymphoma.

Car-T Cells And Immunotherapy As Case Studies

To understand the transformative potential of CAR-T cell therapy, it is essential to explore how this therapy evolved from basic research to clinical application, the successes, challenges, and future directions in this field.

Case Study 1: Car-T Cell Therapy In Acute Lymphoblastic Leukemia (All)

Acute lymphoblastic leukemia (ALL) is a cancer of the blood and bone marrow that affects lymphocytes, a type of white blood cell.

Although treatment for ALL has improved over the years, relapsed or refractory cases remain difficult to manage, particularly in pediatric populations. The introduction of CAR-T cell therapy has led to remarkable results in these patients.

The Development of CAR-T for ALL:
- The first major breakthrough in CAR-T therapy occurred when researchers identified the **CD19 antigen**, which is highly expressed on the surface of B cells, including malignant B cells in ALL.
- By engineering T cells to express a CAR that targets CD19, researchers developed a novel treatment approach that harnesses the power of a patient's immune system to attack and eliminate cancerous B cells.

Clinical Application:
- In clinical trials, CAR-T cell therapies such as **Kymriah** (tisagenlecleucel) demonstrated significant success in

treating relapsed or refractory ALL in both pediatric and adult patients. In one pivotal trial, over 80% of pediatric patients achieved remission after receiving CAR-T cell therapy, with durable responses seen in many patients.

Challenges and Future Directions:
- **Cytokine Release Syndrome (CRS):** A major challenge in CAR-T therapy is the risk of severe side effects, including cytokine release syndrome (CRS), which occurs when the engineered T cells release large amounts of cytokines, leading to severe inflammation and organ damage. Managing CRS requires prompt medical intervention and can limit the applicability of CAR-T therapy.
- **Relapse:** While CAR-T therapy has led to significant responses, some patients may relapse due to the loss of the targeted antigen (CD19) or resistance mechanisms within the tumor. Research is ongoing to address these challenges, including the development of next-generation CAR-T cells targeting multiple antigens.

Case Study 2: Car-T Cell Therapy In Diffuse Large B-Cell Lymphoma (Dlbcl)

Diffuse large B-cell lymphoma (DLBCL) is an aggressive type of non-Hodgkin lymphoma that often presents with poor prognosis, especially in patients whose disease relapses after initial treatment. CAR-T cell therapy has shown promising results in treating relapsed or refractory DLBCL.

The Development of CAR-T for DLBCL:
- Like ALL, researchers focused on the **CD19 antigen** for targeting B cells, leading to the development of CAR-T therapies for DLBCL.
- **Kymriah** and another CAR-T product, **Yescarta** (axicabtagene ciloleucel), have shown promising results in clinical trials for relapsed or refractory DLBCL.

Clinical Application:
- In clinical studies, a significant proportion of patients with relapsed/refractory DLBCL responded to CAR-T therapy. For example, in one trial, nearly 50% of patients who received **Yescarta** achieved complete remission, a notable improvement compared to traditional therapies.
- These therapies offer a potential cure for patients with no other treatment options, transforming the standard of care for relapsed or refractory DLBCL.

Challenges and Future Directions:
- **Tumor Heterogeneity:** Tumor heterogeneity in DLBCL can pose a challenge, as different subtypes of B cells or antigen expression profiles may limit the effectiveness of CAR-T cells.
- **Overcoming Resistance:** Strategies are being explored to overcome resistance mechanisms in CAR-T cell therapy, such as targeting additional antigens, improving CAR constructs, and combining CAR-T with other treatments like immune checkpoint inhibitors.

Immunotherapy In Solid Tumors

While CAR-T cell therapy has had remarkable success in hematologic cancers, the application of immunotherapy to solid tumors, such as lung, breast, and colorectal cancer, has been more challenging. Despite these challenges, advances in immunotherapy have led to promising treatments for certain solid tumors.

Checkpoint Inhibitors

Checkpoint inhibitors, such as **PD-1/PD-L1 inhibitors** and **CTLA-4 inhibitors**, are a class of immunotherapy drugs that target immune checkpoint proteins, thereby allowing the immune system to recognize and attack cancer cells. These drugs have revolutionized the treatment of cancers like melanoma, non-small cell lung cancer (NSCLC), and bladder cancer.

Example: Nivolumab (Opdivo) and **Pembrolizumab (Keytruda)** are PD-1 inhibitors that have shown significant activity in advanced melanoma and lung cancer, respectively.

Tumor-Infiltrating Lymphocytes (TILs)

Another innovative approach to immunotherapy in solid tumors is the use of **tumor-infiltrating lymphocytes (TILs)**. This involves isolating immune cells from a patient's tumor, expanding them in the lab, and then re-infusing them into the patient to enhance the immune response against cancer cells. This strategy has shown success in treating melanoma and other solid tumors.

Challenges In Translational Oncology

Despite the impressive progress in translating research into clinical applications, several challenges persist in oncology:

1. **Tumor Heterogeneity:** The complexity and diversity of tumors make it difficult to develop universal therapies. Tumors may evolve during treatment, leading to resistance and relapse.
2. **Side Effects and Toxicity:** CAR-T cell therapy and immunotherapy can cause severe side effects, such as cytokine release syndrome (CRS) and immune-related adverse events. Managing these side effects is critical for improving patient outcomes.
3. **Cost and Accessibility:** The cost of CAR-T cell therapies and immunotherapies is extremely high, limiting access for many patients. Efforts are underway to reduce costs and expand access to these therapies.
4. **Combination Therapies:** Combining CAR-T therapy with other treatments, such as checkpoint inhibitors or chemotherapy, may enhance efficacy and reduce relapse rates. Ongoing clinical trials are investigating the best ways to combine these therapies.

CHAPTER 11: TRANSLATIONAL MEDICINE IN RARE DISEASES

Translational medicine has opened new frontiers in the treatment of rare diseases, many of which were once considered untreatable.

These diseases, often characterized by their low prevalence, pose unique challenges in both research and treatment development. However, with advances in genomics, gene therapy, and orphan drug development, the landscape for rare disease research and treatment has begun to shift.

Challenges In Rare Disease Research

Rare diseases, defined as conditions that affect fewer than 1 in 2,000 people, encompass a broad array of conditions, many of which are genetic in nature. These diseases often lack effective treatments and present a variety of challenges to researchers, clinicians, and patients alike. Some of the primary challenges in rare disease research include:

1. Limited Patient Population
One of the most significant challenges in rare disease re
search is the limited number of patients, which makes it difficult to conduct large-scale clinical trials.

The scarcity of patients means that recruiting enough participants for randomized controlled trials (RCTs) is often impossible. This leads to difficulties in obtaining statistically significant data, which is essential for proving the efficacy and safety of new treatments.

- **Impact on Trial Design:** Researchers may need to rely on smaller, non-randomized studies or case reports, which can lead to less robust evidence.
- **Potential Solutions:** Patient registries and international collaborations are increasingly being used to gather data across countries and populations. This can help increase the sample size, though it still presents challenges in terms of uniformity and data quality.

2. Limited Understanding of Disease Mechanisms

For many rare diseases, the underlying mechanisms are poorly understood. This is often due to a lack of research funding and attention, as these diseases affect only a small proportion of the population. Without a clear understanding of the molecular and genetic basis of these diseases, it is difficult to develop targeted therapies.

- **Example:** In diseases such as **Duchenne muscular dystrophy (DMD)**, the genetic mutation and its impact on muscle cells were identified, but translating this into effective treatments took decades of research.

3. Regulatory Hurdles

*Regulatory agencies like the **FDA** and **EMA*** face unique challenges when it comes to rare diseases. The small patient populations make it difficult to generate the large amounts of evidence typically required for drug approval.

In addition, *the rarity of these conditions* often means that there is less competition among pharmaceutical companies, which can slow down drug development.

- **Regulatory Flexibility:** Recognizing the unique needs of rare disease treatments, regulatory agencies have introduced special programs, such as orphan drug designations and accelerated approval pathways, to facilitate the development and approval of drugs for rare diseases.

4. High Cost and Limited Market Incentives

The development of treatments for rare diseases is often costly, and pharmaceutical companies may be reluctant to invest heavily in drugs for diseases that affect only a small number of people. The high cost of research, clinical trials, and drug manufacturing means that treatments for rare diseases can be prohibitively expensive.

- **Example: Eteplirsen (Exondys 51)**, a drug developed for **Duchenne muscular dystrophy**, carries a high price tag, often making access difficult for patients.

Advancements In Orphan Drugs And Gene Therapy

Despite these challenges, there have been significant advancements in the field of rare diseases, particularly in the development of orphan drugs and gene therapies.

These breakthroughs are a result of concerted research efforts, improved technologies, and greater collaboration between academic institutions, pharmaceutical companies, and patient advocacy groups.

1. Orphan Drugs

Orphan drugs are pharmaceuticals specifically developed to treat rare diseases. The development of orphan drugs has been supported by various regulatory and financial incentives, including the **Orphan Drug Act** in the U.S. (1983) and similar legislation in other countries.

These incentives include tax credits, research grants, and market exclusivity for a period of time after approval, which help make the development of rare disease treatments more financially viable.

- **Success Stories in Orphan Drug Development:**
  - **Kalydeco (Ivacaftor):** Developed for **cystic fibrosis (CF)**, a genetic disorder caused by mutations in the CFTR gene. Ivacaftor has been shown to significantly improve lung function in patients with specific CFTR mutations, and it marked a major breakthrough in CF treatment. Its approval was expedited under the orphan drug program.
  - **Spinraza (Nusinersen):** Spinraza was approved for the treatment of **spinal muscular atrophy (SMA)**, a genetic disorder that causes progressive muscle weakness. It was one of the first treatments to target the genetic cause of the disease, rather than just managing symptoms. Nusinersen has been shown to improve motor function in patients with SMA.
- **Orphan Drug Designation Process:** Orphan drug designation is granted by the FDA or EMA to encourage the development of treatments for rare diseases. This process provides financial support, but there are still barriers to overcome, such as the high cost of manufacturing and the need for long-term clinical data.

2. Gene Therapy

Gene therapy is rapidly emerging as one of the most promising approaches for treating genetic and rare diseases. Gene therapy aims to correct or replace defective genes responsible for disease, offering potential cures rather than merely treating symptoms.

*Gene therapies can be categorized into several types, including **gene replacement therapy**, **gene editing**, and **gene silencing**.*

- **Gene Replacement Therapy:** This involves introducing a normal copy of a gene into a patient's cells to replace a defective gene. One of the most notable examples of this approach is **Luxturna**, a gene therapy developed to treat **Leber congenital amaurosis (LCA)**, a rare genetic condition that causes blindness. Luxturna delivers a normal copy of the **RPE65 gene** into retinal cells, restoring vision in patients with certain mutations.

- **Gene Editing:** Gene editing technologies, such as **CRISPR-Cas9**, are enabling more precise interventions at the genetic level. By directly editing the patient's genome, researchers can potentially cure diseases caused by single-gene mutations. For example, researchers are exploring CRISPR-based treatments for **sickle cell anemia**, a genetic blood disorder, by editing the defective hemoglobin gene in patients' stem cells.

- **Gene Silencing:** This approach involves turning off or silencing a mutated gene that causes disease. **Spinraza**, mentioned earlier, works by targeting and modifying the **SMN2 gene** in patients with SMA, increasing the production of the survival motor neuron protein and slowing the progression of the disease.

- **Challenges in Gene Therapy for Rare Diseases:** Although gene therapy holds immense promise, it faces challenges such as high costs, delivery methods, and long-term safety. Ensuring that the delivered genes integrate correctly into the patient's DNA without causing side effects such as cancer is a critical hurdle that needs to be addressed. Additionally, the high cost of gene therapies has raised concerns about accessibility, particularly for rare diseases with small patient populations.

Collaborations And Global Efforts

The development of therapies for rare diseases often requires collaboration across multiple sectors.

Research institutions, biotech companies, patient advocacy groups, and regulatory agencies must work together to overcome the unique challenges posed by rare diseases.

- **Global Partnerships:** International collaborations, such as the **International Rare Diseases Research Consortium (IRDiRC)**, aim to accelerate the development of new treatments for rare diseases by bringing together researchers and funding organizations from around the world.

- **Patient Advocacy:** Patient advocacy groups play a crucial role in driving research efforts for rare diseases. They help raise awareness, fund research, and provide crucial insights into the lived experience of patients, ensuring that treatment development is patient-centered.

CHAPTER 12: TRANSLATIONAL MEDICINE IN INFECTIOUS DISEASES

Infectious diseases remain a major global health threat, with emerging and re-emerging pathogens constantly challenging medical and public health systems.

Translational medicine plays a crucial role in the development of new therapies, vaccines, and diagnostic tools that bridge the gap between laboratory research and patient care. The COVID-19 pandemic served as a stark reminder of the importance of rapid translational research and has significantly accelerated the development of innovative therapeutic approaches.

Lessons From Covid-19 Vaccine Development

The rapid development and deployment of COVID-19 vaccines marked a pivotal moment in translational medicine. *The unprecedented speed* with which safe and effective vaccines were developed showcased the potential of translational research in infectious diseases. Several key lessons emerged from the COVID-19 vaccine development process, each of which can inform future approaches to combating infectious diseases:

1. Collaborative Efforts Across Sectors

One of the most striking lessons from COVID-19 vaccine development was the power of collaboration between academic institutions, private industry, governments, and nongovernmental organizations. This multi-sector collaboration allowed for the sharing of resources, expertise, and data, which accelerated the development process.

- **Example:** The partnership between **Pfizer-BioNTech** and **Moderna** led to the rapid development of mRNA-based vaccines, leveraging years of prior research in vaccine technology and biotechnology. Both companies had been working on mRNA vaccines for other diseases (such as cancer and influenza) prior to the pandemic, which enabled them to pivot quickly when the novel coronavirus emerged.
- **Public-Private Partnerships:** The U.S. government's **Operation Warp Speed** played a key role in expediting the vaccine development process by providing significant funding and logistical support to vaccine developers. This demonstrated the importance of government support in catalyzing the rapid translation of research into public health interventions.

2. Innovation In Vaccine Platforms

The COVID-19 vaccines utilized innovative technologies that had not previously been used on such a large scale. These platforms include mRNA vaccines, viral vector vaccines, and protein subunit vaccines.

- **mRNA Vaccines (Pfizer-BioNTech and Moderna):** mRNA technology allows for the development of vaccines that instruct cells to produce a piece of the viral spike protein, which then triggers an immune response. This platform had been in development for several years, but the pandemic provided the impetus for its first major real-world application. mRNA vaccines were developed in record time, offering high efficacy and safety.

- **Viral Vector Vaccines (Oxford-AstraZeneca and Johnson & Johnson):** Viral vector vaccines use harmless viruses (such as adenovirus) to deliver genetic material encoding a viral antigen into cells. This approach was also proven effective and provided an alternative to mRNA-based vaccines.
- **Protein Subunit Vaccines (Novavax):** This platform involves using pieces of the virus (such as the spike protein) to stimulate an immune response. The **Novavax** vaccine is an example of a protein subunit vaccine that showed promise in clinical trials.

3. Importance Of Prior Research And Preparedness

The speed of COVID-19 vaccine development was made possible by years of prior research into coronaviruses and vaccine technologies. The development of **SARS-CoV-2 vaccines** benefited from previous work on **SARS-CoV** (2003) and **MERS-CoV** (2012), as well as ongoing research into other respiratory viruses like the flu.

- **Vaccine Platforms for Other Diseases:** Researchers had already developed and tested mRNA vaccines for other diseases, such as **Zika virus** and **HIV**, allowing for a quicker adaptation when SARS-CoV-2 emerged.
- **Global Vaccine Network:** The establishment of global networks like **GAVI, the Vaccine Alliance**, and the **Coalition for Epidemic Preparedness Innovations (CEPI)** supported early research into vaccines and diagnostics, providing a framework for rapid action.

4. Rapid Clinical Trials And Regulatory Flexibility

The regulatory landscape surrounding vaccine development was also transformed during the COVID-19 pandemic. Regulatory agencies like the **FDA, EMA**, and **WHO** offered expedited pathways for emergency use authorization (EUA) to allow for faster access to life-saving treatments.

- **Adaptive Trial Designs:** Many of the clinical trials for COVID-19 vaccines employed **adaptive trial designs**, which allowed researchers to modify trials as they progressed based on real-time data. This approach was critical in assessing the safety and efficacy of vaccines in different populations and settings.
- **Emergency Use Authorization (EUA):** Under EUA, regulatory agencies granted temporary approval for the use of vaccines before completing full-scale, long-term studies, based on promising early results. This flexibility in regulatory pathways allowed for rapid deployment without compromising patient safety.

Translating Research Into Pandemic Preparedness

The lessons learned from the rapid development of COVID-19 vaccines underscore the importance of preparedness and infrastructure in the context of infectious disease outbreaks.

Translational medicine plays a critical role in ensuring that research is not only conducted but also translated into effective public health interventions that can be deployed rapidly in the face of an emerging pandemic.

Some key strategies for improving pandemic preparedness include:

1. Strengthening Global Surveillance Systems

A key factor in the rapid response to COVID-19 was the **global surveillance** and early identification of the virus. Early detection allows for quicker responses and more effective containment measures.

- **Example:** The **Global Influenza Surveillance and Response System (GISRS)**, managed by the **WHO**, provided a template for how surveillance systems

can detect novel viruses and inform the development of vaccines and treatments. Expanding and strengthening these systems is essential for future pandemic preparedness.
- **Next-Generation Surveillance Tools:** Leveraging **big data**, **artificial intelligence (AI)**, and **machine learning (ML)** can help enhance surveillance systems to identify emerging threats more rapidly. These tools can analyze vast amounts of data, from clinical cases to genomic sequences, to detect potential outbreaks early.

2. Rapid Response Platforms

The development of rapid-response platforms, such as mRNA vaccine technology, must be further accelerated and institutionalized for future pandemics. These platforms need to be adaptable to different pathogens, allowing for the swift deployment of vaccines and therapeutics once a new virus is identified.

- **Platform Technologies:** Building on the success of COVID-19 mRNA vaccines, researchers are exploring mRNA vaccine platforms for diseases such as **Zika virus**, **HIV**, and **influenza**. These platforms could be rapidly adapted to new pathogens in the future, reducing the time needed for vaccine development.

3. Global Collaboration And Data Sharing

The COVID-19 pandemic highlighted the importance of international collaboration in research, vaccine development, and distribution. Countries and organizations must work together to share data, resources, and expertise to address global health crises.

- **Example:** The **COVAX initiative**, aimed at equitable global access to COVID-19 vaccines, emphasized

the need for collaboration between public health organizations, governments, and vaccine manufacturers to ensure vaccines were distributed fairly to low- and middle-income countries.
- **International Research Consortia:** Future pandemic preparedness should include the formation of international research consortia that can pool resources and knowledge to address infectious disease threats quickly.

4. Preparedness Beyond Vaccines

While vaccines are a critical tool in preventing pandemics, they must be part of a broader, more comprehensive preparedness plan that includes diagnostics, therapeutics, and public health infrastructure.

- **Diagnostics:** Rapid diagnostic tests are essential for identifying infections early and containing outbreaks. The success of COVID-19 diagnostic testing, including **PCR** and **antigen tests**, should be leveraged to develop broader diagnostic networks for future pandemics.
- **Therapeutics:** In addition to vaccines, research into antiviral drugs and other therapies must be accelerated. Treatments like **remdesivir** and **monoclonal antibodies** have shown promise for COVID-19, but more work is needed to develop effective antiviral therapies for future pathogens.

5. Ethical And Equity Considerations

Equitable distribution of vaccines, therapies, and diagnostics remains one of the greatest challenges in global pandemic preparedness.

The COVID-19 pandemic demonstrated the disparities in access to healthcare, with high-income countries having faster access to vaccines and therapeutics compared to low- and middle-income countries.

- **Global Health Equity:** Future pandemic preparedness strategies must ensure that all populations, particularly the most vulnerable, have equal access to life-saving interventions. This requires not only ensuring global supply chains but also addressing political and economic barriers to healthcare access.

CHAPTER 13: EMERGING TRENDS IN TRANSLATIONAL MEDICINE

The field of translational medicine is constantly evolving, driven by rapid advancements in technology, research, and an ever-deepening understanding of human biology. As we move into the future, new tools, strategies, and paradigms are shaping the way research is conducted and how it translates into patient care.

Among the most significant emerging trends in translational medicine are the growing roles of digital health technologies, artificial intelligence (AI), and machine learning (ML), which have the potential to revolutionize the way we understand, diagnose, and treat diseases.

Role Of Digital Health Technologies

Digital health technologies are rapidly transforming the landscape of healthcare by enabling the continuous monitoring of patient health, facilitating remote care, and supporting personalized treatment approaches. These technologies are increasingly integrated into translational research, creating new opportunities to bridge the gap between laboratory discoveries and clinical application. Some of the most notable digital health technologies include:

1. Wearables And Mobile Health Devices

Wearables, such as fitness trackers, smartwatches, and wearable ECG monitors, are revolutionizing the way health data is collected and analyzed. These devices can track a wide range of physiological parameters in real-time, such as heart rate, blood pressure, physical activity, sleep patterns, and even glucose levels. This continuous data collection opens new avenues for both research and patient care, *allowing for*:

- **Personalized Treatment:** Real-time health data can provide insights into how a patient is responding to treatment, enabling clinicians to adjust medications and interventions promptly.
- **Early Detection:** Wearables can help identify changes in a patient's condition long before symptoms appear, allowing for earlier interventions and potentially better outcomes.
- **Clinical Trials:** Wearable devices can be used in clinical trials to monitor participants' health remotely, reducing the need for frequent hospital visits and improving the accessibility and inclusivity of trials.

2. Telemedicine And Remote Patient Monitoring

The COVID-19 pandemic accelerated the adoption of telemedicine, which has now become an essential component of healthcare delivery. Telemedicine allows patients to consult with healthcare providers remotely, reducing the barriers to care, especially for those in rural or underserved areas.

In translational medicine, telemedicine and remote patient monitoring technologies enable:

- **Enhanced Access to Care:** Patients in remote locations can access specialists and participate in clinical trials without needing to travel long distances.
- **Continuous Data Collection:** Through remote monitoring tools, data on patient health can be gathered continuously, providing more detailed insights into disease progression and treatment efficacy.

- **Patient Engagement:** Telemedicine platforms can facilitate communication between patients and researchers, ensuring that participants in clinical trials remain engaged and informed.

3. Digital Therapeutics And Virtual Interventions

Digital therapeutics are evidence-based interventions delivered through software or digital platforms to prevent, manage, or treat medical conditions. These therapies can be particularly useful in the management of chronic diseases, such as diabetes, heart disease, and mental health conditions.

Digital therapeutics are increasingly incorporated into translational medicine for:

- **Behavioral Health:** Virtual therapies for mental health conditions, such as cognitive behavioral therapy (CBT) apps, provide a non-invasive treatment option that can be tailored to individual needs and accessed conveniently.
- **Chronic Disease Management:** Digital tools designed to help patients manage chronic conditions—such as diabetes apps that track blood sugar levels—can lead to better disease management and improved patient outcomes.
- **Clinical Trials:** Digital therapeutics are increasingly being tested in clinical trials as an adjunct or alternative to traditional treatments, especially in areas like neurology, oncology, and mental health.

Integration Of Artificial Intelligence And Machine

Learning

Artificial intelligence (AI) and machine learning (ML) are two transformative technologies that are playing an increasingly prominent role in translational medicine. These tools can process vast amounts of data, recognize patterns, and make predictions that would be impossible for humans to achieve on their own.

Their integration into translational research and clinical practice is poised to accelerate discoveries, improve decision-making, and create more personalized treatment plans.

1. Ai In Drug Discovery And Development

AI and ML are revolutionizing the process of drug discovery by enabling the analysis of large datasets, identifying potential drug candidates, and predicting how new compounds will behave in the human body. This can significantly reduce the time and cost involved in developing new treatments.

AI's applications in drug discovery include:

- **Target Identification:** Machine learning algorithms can sift through vast amounts of biological data to identify potential targets for new drugs. This helps researchers focus their efforts on the most promising areas of research.
- **Drug Screening:** AI models can predict which compounds are most likely to interact with specific disease targets, speeding up the process of drug screening and reducing the need for lengthy and expensive laboratory testing.
- **Drug Repurposing:** AI can analyze existing drugs to identify new uses for them, accelerating the availability of treatments for diseases that currently lack effective therapies.

2. Ai In Diagnostics And Personalized Medicine

AI's ability to analyze complex patterns in data has made it an invaluable tool in the development of diagnostic technologies. Machine learning algorithms can process medical imaging data, genomic data, and patient health records to identify disease patterns that may not be visible to the human eye, *leading to:*

- **Enhanced Diagnostics:** AI-powered tools are already being used to analyze medical imaging (such as MRIs and CT scans) for signs of diseases like cancer, stroke, and neurodegenerative disorders. These tools can provide early detection of conditions, improving treatment outcomes.
- **Predictive Analytics:** By integrating AI with electronic health records, researchers and clinicians can use predictive analytics to anticipate disease progression, predict treatment responses, and personalize treatment plans for patients based on their unique genetic and health profiles.
- **Precision Medicine:** AI-driven approaches enable the tailoring of treatments to individual patients, optimizing drug regimens and dosages for each person's specific genetic makeup, lifestyle, and health history. This can greatly enhance the effectiveness of treatments while minimizing side effects.

3. Ai In Clinical Trials

AI and ML are transforming clinical trial design and management by making it easier to recruit participants, monitor their health in real-time, and analyze outcomes.

AI can improve clinical trials in several key areas:

- **Patient Recruitment:** AI algorithms can identify

eligible participants more quickly by analyzing patient databases and matching them with appropriate trials. This can increase recruitment rates and ensure that trials are conducted more efficiently.

- **Monitoring and Data Analysis:** AI tools can monitor patient health remotely during trials, ensuring that side effects or adverse events are detected early. Additionally, AI can analyze trial data more quickly than traditional methods, identifying trends and outcomes that might otherwise go unnoticed.
- **Adaptive Trials:** AI can facilitate the use of adaptive trial designs, where treatment protocols can be adjusted in real-time based on emerging data. This allows for more flexible, responsive trials that can be more efficient and provide better insights.

4. Ai In Health Systems And Decision Support

Beyond the lab and clinical trial setting, AI is becoming an integral part of healthcare systems. AI-powered decision support systems help healthcare providers make more informed decisions about patient care. These systems can integrate data from multiple sources—such as patient records, clinical guidelines, and research data—and offer actionable insights.

- **Clinical Decision Support:** AI tools can provide clinicians with real-time recommendations for diagnosis and treatment based on the patient's unique clinical data. This can help reduce diagnostic errors, improve treatment efficacy, and ensure that patients receive the best possible care.
- **Population Health Management:** AI can analyze health trends across populations, identifying patterns in disease prevalence, treatment outcomes, and patient behavior. This can help healthcare providers and

policymakers allocate resources more effectively and design interventions that target the most at-risk populations.

CHAPTER 14: BUILDING A SUSTAINABLE FUTURE

As translational medicine continues to evolve, it is essential to build a sustainable framework that not only accelerates scientific discoveries but also ensures these advances benefit society in the long term.

For translational medicine to achieve its full potential, we must focus on educating the next generation of researchers, developing innovative strategies for funding, and establishing policies that support a collaborative, interdisciplinary, and inclusive environment.

Educating The Next Generation Of Researchers

The future of translational medicine relies heavily on the development of a skilled, multidisciplinary workforce capable of navigating the complexities of modern medical research and patient care. Building a pipeline of talented researchers, clinicians, and innovators is essential for the continued advancement of the field.

This requires a comprehensive approach to education that spans undergraduate to postdoctoral levels and includes a variety of training opportunities tailored to the unique demands of translational research.

1. Interdisciplinary Training Programs

Translational medicine operates at the intersection of basic science, clinical research, and patient care. Therefore, fostering interdisciplinary training is key to ensuring that future researchers can collaborate effectively across different fields. *This involves:*

- **Collaborative Curricula:** Developing academic programs that encourage students from diverse backgrounds—such as biology, engineering, computer science, and medicine—to work together. These programs can be designed to integrate foundational knowledge in each discipline while also emphasizing the practical application of that knowledge to real-world healthcare challenges.
- **Dual-Degree Programs:** Offering dual-degree programs that allow students to earn both medical and scientific research degrees (e.g., MD/PhD programs). These programs help cultivate researchers who have a deep understanding of both clinical practice and the scientific research process, which is crucial for bridging the gap between laboratory discoveries and patient care.
- **Collaborations with Industry and Government:** Universities should partner with pharmaceutical companies, biotech firms, and government organizations to provide students with exposure to real-world challenges in translational medicine. These partnerships can also help create internship and fellowship opportunities where students can gain hands-on experience working on innovative projects.

2. Specialized Training For Early-Career Researchers

While foundational training is critical, it is equally important to provide early-career researchers with the tools they need to succeed in translational medicine.

Specialized training programs can include:

- **Clinical-Research Fellowships:** These programs offer researchers who are trained in basic science an opportunity to work in clinical settings and gain hands-on experience in the translation of research into therapies and interventions. This helps build a bridge between laboratory work and patient care, which is essential for translating discoveries into practice.
- **Mentorship Programs:** Establishing mentorship programs that pair early-career researchers with experienced scientists and clinicians is crucial for nurturing new talent. Mentorship helps young researchers develop the necessary skills to navigate complex translational projects, including grant writing, project management, and interdisciplinary collaboration.
- **Leadership and Communication Skills:** As translational medicine requires effective communication between multiple stakeholders (researchers, clinicians, patients, regulatory agencies, and policymakers), training in leadership, communication, and public engagement should be an integral part of a researcher's education.

3. Lifelong Learning And Continuous Professional Development

Given the rapid pace of technological advances in translational medicine, it is important to encourage lifelong learning and continuous professional development. Researchers must stay up-to-date with the latest developments in areas such as genomics, big data, AI, and new therapeutic approaches.

This can be achieved through:

- **Workshops and Conferences:** Regular workshops, seminars, and conferences should be held to expose researchers to the latest advancements in the field and allow for networking with other professionals across disciplines.
- **Online Learning Platforms:** Universities and research organizations can also leverage online platforms to offer courses and webinars focused on emerging topics in translational medicine, ensuring that professionals can access flexible learning opportunities as they advance in their careers.

Policy Recommendations To Foster Translational Medicine

While the scientific and educational components of translational medicine are crucial, supportive policies are essential to foster a robust research environment and ensure that innovations reach patients in a timely and ethical manner.

Governments, regulatory agencies, and institutions need to implement policies that encourage collaboration, enhance funding opportunities, and streamline the path from research to clinical application.

1. Increase Funding For Translational Research

One of the biggest challenges in translational medicine is securing adequate funding to support research across the various stages of development, from discovery through to clinical trials and implementation.

Governments, private institutions, and philanthropic organizations should prioritize funding for translational research by:

- **Targeted Research Grants:** Allocating funds

specifically for translational medicine initiatives that address high-priority public health challenges. These grants should encourage interdisciplinary projects and foster collaborations between academic researchers, clinicians, and industry partners.

- **Long-term Investment:** Translational research can be expensive and time-consuming, with uncertain outcomes. Governments and private investors should be willing to commit to long-term funding for projects that have the potential to transform healthcare. This includes supporting early-stage research as well as later phases, such as clinical trials and regulatory approval.
- **Tax Incentives and Subsidies for Industry Collaboration:** Offering tax incentives and subsidies for private companies, including biotech and pharmaceutical firms, to invest in translational medicine projects can stimulate innovation and accelerate the development of new treatments.

2. Streamline Regulatory Processes

Regulatory hurdles can slow down the progress of translating research into patient care. Governments and regulatory agencies should implement policies that streamline the approval processes for new therapies, diagnostics, and medical devices, without compromising patient safety.

Recommendations include:

- **Regulatory Pathway Optimization:** Governments and regulatory bodies (such as the FDA and EMA) should work together to create clear, efficient regulatory pathways for novel therapies that have the potential to address unmet medical needs. This may involve the creation of specialized regulatory pathways for

breakthrough therapies and accelerated approval processes.
- **Adaptive Trials:** Regulatory agencies should encourage the use of adaptive trial designs that allow for adjustments to be made to ongoing clinical trials based on emerging data. This flexibility can speed up the process of testing and refining new treatments.
- **Global Regulatory Harmonization:** As translational research becomes increasingly global, it is crucial to harmonize regulatory standards across different regions. This would allow for smoother international collaboration and faster access to new therapies across borders.

3. Foster Public-Private Partnerships

Public-private partnerships (PPPs) play a crucial role in advancing translational medicine by combining the resources and expertise of the public and private sectors. Governments should support the establishment of PPPs to:

- **Facilitate Knowledge Sharing:** PPPs can promote the exchange of knowledge and expertise between academic researchers, healthcare providers, and industry stakeholders, fostering innovation and accelerating the development of new therapies.
- **Enhance Access to Resources:** Private sector involvement in public research projects can provide access to financial resources, infrastructure, and advanced technologies that may not otherwise be available in academic or government research settings.
- **Increase Patient-Centric Research:** By involving patients in the design and implementation of research projects, PPPs can ensure that the research is aligned with the real-world needs of patients, improving the

likelihood of successful outcomes.

4. Strengthen Ethics And Oversight Frameworks

As translational medicine often involves high-stakes clinical trials, gene therapies, and novel treatment modalities, ensuring ethical conduct is paramount. Governments and institutions should strengthen ethical oversight by:

- **Robust Ethical Review Processes:** Institutional Review Boards (IRBs) and Ethics Committees should be equipped with the resources and expertise to evaluate the ethical implications of translational research, ensuring that research involving human participants is conducted safely and with full informed consent.
- **Patient-Centered Policies:** Policies should prioritize the rights and welfare of patients involved in clinical trials, ensuring that they are fully informed of the risks and benefits of participating in research. Furthermore, patient privacy and data security must be safeguarded.
- **Addressing Health Inequities:** Policies should encourage the inclusion of diverse populations in clinical research to ensure that new therapies are effective across all demographic groups. This includes addressing the unique needs of underserved populations, such as those from rural areas or lower-income communities.

CHAPTER 15: CONCLUSION AND CALL TO ACTION

Translational medicine stands at the crossroads of scientific discovery and patient care, with the potential to revolutionize healthcare and create transformative therapies that address some of the world's most pressing medical challenges. Over the course of this book, we have explored the journey from basic research to clinical application, highlighting the importance of collaboration, ethics, technology, and funding in bridging the gap between the laboratory bench and the patient's bedside. As we move forward, the need for continuous innovation, collaboration, and global cooperation remains more pressing than ever.

The Need For Continuous Innovation

Translational medicine is a dynamic and ever-evolving field that thrives on innovation. The speed at which scientific advancements are occurring—particularly in genomics, artificial intelligence, and personalized medicine—requires constant adaptation to new discoveries, technologies, and approaches.

As the healthcare landscape continues to change, the need for continuous innovation in the realm of translational medicine has never been more crucial.

1. Pushing The Boundaries Of Scientific Discovery

The frontier of translational medicine lies at the intersection of cutting-edge science and clinical application. With every breakthrough in fields such as genomics, gene therapy, and immunotherapy, new possibilities emerge for treating previously untreatable conditions. However, to realize the full potential of these advancements, researchers must continue pushing the boundaries of what is possible. This includes:

- **Expanding the Scope of Research:** While much of the current focus in translational medicine has been on cancer, infectious diseases, and rare diseases, there is an urgent need to apply these innovations to a broader range of health challenges. Chronic conditions such as diabetes, cardiovascular diseases, and neurodegenerative disorders require novel approaches that can be accelerated through translational research.
- **Leveraging Interdisciplinary Collaboration:** The complexities of modern diseases require expertise from a diverse range of disciplines. Encouraging collaboration between researchers, clinicians, engineers, data scientists, and patients will drive the development of multifaceted solutions that address the root causes of diseases rather than just their symptoms.
- **Harnessing New Technologies:** The role of artificial intelligence, machine learning, and big data cannot be overstated in the context of translational medicine. These technologies hold the power to analyze vast datasets, predict disease outcomes, and tailor personalized treatment strategies that can significantly improve patient outcomes. Researchers must continue to innovate with these tools to unlock their full potential in medicine.

2. Addressing The Complexity Of Human Health

Human health is inherently complex, and diseases rarely fit neatly into categories. Translational medicine must evolve to tackle these complexities, focusing not only on curing diseases but also on preventing them, improving quality of life, and addressing social determinants of health.

- **Holistic Approaches to Healthcare:** To achieve true patient-centered care, translational medicine must go beyond individual therapies and consider the broader context of health, including genetics, environment, lifestyle, and social factors. Research must integrate these elements to create personalized, preventive care strategies.
- **Patient-Reported Outcomes:** Incorporating patient voices into research design and treatment protocols is essential. Patient-reported outcomes (PROs) can provide valuable insights into how treatments impact patients' quality of life, and these should be integrated into clinical trials and post-market surveillance.

Bridging Global Gaps In Research And Patient Care

While translational medicine has made tremendous strides, there are still significant gaps in research and patient care, particularly in low- and middle-income countries (LMICs) and underserved communities.

The benefits of scientific discoveries must be made accessible to all, not just those in wealthy or resource-rich regions. Bridging these global gaps requires both a commitment to equity and a strategic approach to global collaboration.

1. Equitable Access to Healthcare Innovations

The success of translational medicine hinges on ensuring that innovations in research and treatment are accessible to all patients, regardless of their geographical location, socioeconomic status, or ethnicity. This requires:

- **Affordable Access to New Therapies:** High-cost therapies, especially those in fields like gene therapy and personalized medicine, must be made affordable and accessible to patients across the globe. This involves not only lowering the costs of these treatments but also improving healthcare infrastructure and delivery in underserved regions.

- **Global Distribution Networks:** Efficient global distribution networks are necessary to ensure that life-saving drugs, vaccines, and medical technologies reach people in all parts of the world. Partnerships between governments, NGOs, and the private sector can help facilitate this process.
- **Addressing Health Inequities:** It is essential to tackle health disparities by ensuring that research in translational medicine includes diverse populations, particularly those from underrepresented regions and communities. This includes both genetic diversity and the consideration of social, economic, and cultural factors that influence health outcomes.

2. Strengthening Global Research Collaboration

The future of translational medicine depends on fostering international cooperation. By sharing knowledge, resources, and expertise, researchers can accelerate the development of treatments and solutions that benefit people worldwide.

Strategies for strengthening global research collaboration include:

- **International Research Consortia:** Governments, academic institutions, and industry partners should collaborate on large-scale international research consortia to address global health challenges. By pooling resources and expertise, these partnerships can tackle diseases that disproportionately affect populations in different parts of the world, such as malaria, tuberculosis, and neglected tropical diseases.
- **Data Sharing and Open Science:** The principles of open

science and data sharing are essential for accelerating progress in translational medicine. By creating open-access platforms where researchers can freely share data, findings, and methodologies, we can reduce redundancy, enhance collaboration, and expedite discoveries. This openness is particularly vital for ensuring that researchers from all corners of the globe can contribute to and benefit from global scientific advancements.

- **Capacity Building in Low-Resource Settings:** One of the most important aspects of global collaboration is building research capacity in low- and middle-income countries. This can be achieved through international partnerships that provide training, resources, and infrastructure to enable local researchers to conduct high-quality translational research. Such initiatives not only improve global healthcare but also empower local communities and researchers to take ownership of their own health challenges.

A Call To Action: Moving Forward Together

The future of translational medicine is filled with promise, but realizing this promise requires concerted action from all stakeholders involved in the process—from researchers and clinicians to policymakers and patients.

To move forward, we must embrace the following principles:

- **Collaboration and Interdisciplinary Partnerships:** Translational medicine thrives on collaboration. Researchers, clinicians, industry leaders, and patients must work together to identify and solve pressing healthcare challenges. Embracing diversity in expertise and perspectives will lead to more innovative solutions and ensure that no one is left behind.

- **Sustained Investment and Funding:** Translational research requires significant financial investment, and governments, private companies, and philanthropists must continue to prioritize funding for the translation of research into practice. By investing in both early-stage research and the later phases of clinical trials and implementation, we can bring new treatments to market faster and more efficiently.
- **Global Cooperation for Global Health:** The challenges facing healthcare are not confined to any one country or region. To tackle the global health crises of the future, we must work together across borders, cultures, and disciplines. This means sharing data, resources, and expertise to accelerate research and ensure that life-saving therapies reach everyone in need.
- **Patient-Centered Focus:** Translational medicine must always prioritize the needs and voices of patients. By integrating patient feedback, ensuring equitable access to healthcare, and improving health outcomes, we can create a healthcare system that truly benefits everyone.

APPENDIX

Glossary Of Key Terms

A glossary of key terms can serve as a useful reference for readers unfamiliar with some of the specialized terminology used in translational medicine. This section will define important concepts and terms that are commonly encountered in the field, ensuring that the book is accessible to readers of all backgrounds.

1. **Translational Medicine**
   The process of applying discoveries made in the laboratory to develop new treatments and therapies for patients. It is the bridge between basic scientific research and clinical application, with the goal of improving patient care.

2. **Basic Research (T0)**
   Fundamental scientific investigations aimed at understanding biological processes at the molecular, cellular, and genetic levels. This research typically does not have immediate clinical applications but lays the groundwork for future developments.

3. **Preclinical Research (T1)**
   Research conducted in the laboratory or using animal models to test new therapies, drugs, or medical devices before they are used in humans.

4. **Clinical Research (T2)**
   Research that involves testing interventions in human subjects, usually in controlled clinical trials, to assess their safety and efficacy.

5. **Clinical Trials (T3)**
   Rigorous studies involving human participants that evaluate the safety, dosage, and therapeutic effects of new interventions, therapies, or drugs.

6. **Implementation Science (T4)**
   The study of methods to promote the adoption of evidence-based practices and interventions into everyday clinical care to improve patient outcomes and healthcare delivery.

7. **Personalized Medicine**
   An approach to medical treatment and healthcare that tailors interventions to individual patients based on genetic, environmental, and lifestyle factors.

8. **Biomarkers**
   Biological indicators (usually proteins, genes, or metabolites) that are measured to assess the presence or severity of disease, predict the response to treatment, or monitor the progress of a disease.

9. **Pharmacogenomics**
   The study of how genes influence an individual's response to drugs. This is key to the development of personalized therapies that are more effective and have fewer side effects.

10. **Regulatory Agencies**
    Governmental organizations responsible for overseeing the safety, efficacy, and approval of medical products. The **FDA** (Food and Drug Administration) in the U.S. and the **EMA** (European Medicines Agency) are two major regulatory bodies.

11. **Orphan Drugs**
    Medications developed to treat rare diseases, often with a small patient population. Due to their limited market, the development of orphan drugs is typically incentivized by special regulatory policies.

12. **Gene Therapy**
    A technique that involves modifying a person's genes to treat or cure diseases by replacing defective genes with healthy ones or altering genes to improve their function.

13. **Biologics**
    A category of treatments derived from living organisms, such as monoclonal antibodies, vaccines, or gene therapies, which are used to treat various diseases, including cancers and autoimmune disorders.

14. **Immunotherapy**
    A treatment that uses the body's immune system to fight diseases such as cancer. It can involve stimulating the immune system or administering engineered immune cells to target and destroy cancer cells.

15. **Fast-Track Approval**
    A designation by the FDA or other regulatory agencies that expedites the development and review of drugs or treatments that address unmet medical needs for serious or life-threatening conditions.

16. **Biomarker Discovery**
    The identification of biological markers that can be used to predict the onset of a disease, assess the severity of the disease, or monitor treatment responses.

17. **Ethical Oversight**
    The process of ensuring that clinical trials and other medical research are conducted ethically, with proper consideration for participant safety, informed consent, and privacy.

18. **Public-Private Partnerships (PPPs)**
    Collaborative initiatives between government bodies,

academic institutions, and private sector companies designed to share resources, knowledge, and expertise to advance translational medicine and bring new treatments to market.

Recommended Reading And Resources

To deepen your understanding of translational medicine and explore further resources, the following books, journals, websites, and organizations are highly recommended:

Books:

1. **"Translational Medicine: Tools and Techniques" by Michael L. Brown** This book offers an in-depth look at the tools, technologies, and methodologies that support the transition of basic science discoveries into clinical applications.

2. **"Principles of Translational Science in Medicine" by M. M. Gottesman** A comprehensive guide that explores the fundamental principles of translational science, discussing how scientific discoveries are turned into treatments and therapies.

3. **"The Translational Medicine Handbook: From the Bench to the Bedside" by Alan R. Shalev** A practical guide that outlines key stages of the translational research process, with case studies and examples from a variety of therapeutic areas.

4. **"Translational Medicine and Drug Discovery: Targeted Therapy and Personalized Medicine" by Alice C. S. Yang** A resource focused on the intersection of translational research, drug discovery, and personalized medicine, with emphasis on cancer and genetic disorders.

Journals:

1. **Translational Medicine Communications**
A leading journal that publishes high-quality research articles on all aspects of translational medicine, from laboratory studies to clinical applications and public health.

2. **Nature Translational Medicine**
   This journal covers the latest developments in translating scientific discoveries into clinical therapies, with articles on clinical trials, molecular medicine, and healthcare innovation.

3. **Journal of Translational Medicine**
   A peer-reviewed journal that publishes research on the application of scientific discoveries to clinical practice, including clinical trials, epidemiology, and translational research.

4. **Clinical Translational Science**
   A journal focusing on research that advances the process of translating basic science into clinical practices, including new therapeutic strategies and technologies.

Websites:

1. **National Institutes of Health (NIH) – Translational Medicine**
   The NIH's dedicated webpage on translational medicine, featuring resources, funding opportunities, and links to major research initiatives in translational science.
   Website: www.nih.gov

2. **European Medicines Agency (EMA)**
   Provides information about regulatory processes, guidelines, and approvals in the context of translational medicine in Europe.
   Website: www.ema.europa.eu

3. **FDA – Translational Medicine**
   The U.S. FDA's website on translational medicine, offering resources on drug development, regulatory pathways, and clinical trials.
   Website: www.fda.gov

4. **Open Science Framework**

A platform for collaboration and sharing research data, publications, and tools across the scientific community.
Website: www.osf.io

Organizations:

1. **The Translational Medicine Society (TMS)**
   A global organization dedicated to the advancement of translational research and its application to clinical medicine. TMS provides educational resources, networking opportunities, and conferences.
   Website: www.translationalmedicine.org

2. **The Clinical and Translational Science Award (CTSA) Program**
   Funded by the NIH, this program supports collaborative initiatives that bridge the gap between scientific discoveries and clinical applications.
   Website: www.ctsaweb.org

3. **World Health Organization (WHO) – Translational Research**
   The WHO offers guidance on the application of translational medicine in global health initiatives, focusing on areas like infectious diseases and non-communicable diseases.
   Website: www.who.int

4. **Orphan Drug Consortium**
   An organization that supports the development of orphan drugs for rare diseases, helping researchers navigate regulatory hurdles and gain access to funding.
   Website: www.orphan-drug.org

ABOUT THE AUTHOR

Dr Essam Abdelhakim

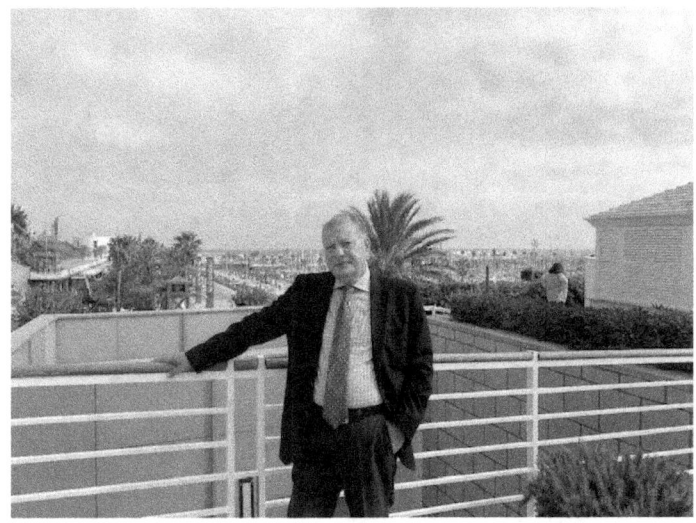

Senior Investigator and Expert in Clinical research

www.ingramcontent.com/pod-product-compliance
Lightning Source LLC
Chambersburg PA
CBHW071036240526
45469CB00006BD/2234